AF487132

PATH TO WELLNESS

PATH TO WELLNESS

CARMEN WILDE

CONTENTS

Copyright © 2024 by Carmen Wilde
All rights reserved. No part of this book may be reproduced in any manner whatsoever without written permission except in the case of brief quotations embodied in critical articles and reviews.
First Printing, 2024

Introduction

Purpose: This book is designed to be a comprehensive guide that leads readers through the essential steps to achieve and maintain wellness. With practical advice, scientific insights, and personal anecdotes, "Path to Wellness" will help readers understand the vital aspects of health and how to integrate them into their daily lives.

About the Author: Carmen Wilde is a dedicated Nurse Practitioner with over 15 years of experience in promoting wellness and preventive care. Carmen's commitment to improving patient outcomes and fostering holistic health approaches has established her as a trusted voice in the healthcare community. With a passion for educating and empowering individuals, she brings a wealth of knowledge and a compassionate approach to wellness.

Defining Wellness: Wellness is a holistic concept that encompasses physical, mental, and emotional health. It's about creating a balanced life where all aspects of well-being are nurtured. This book will explore these dimensions and provide actionable steps to help you achieve a harmonious and fulfilling life.

Do you want to flesh out any more sections?

Chapter 1:
Understanding Wellness

Defining Wellness

To embark on a journey towards wellness, we first need to understand what it truly means. Wellness is often mistakenly equated with physical health alone, but it encompasses so much more. It is a dynamic, multifaceted state that combines physical, mental, emotional, social, and spiritual well-being. Think of it as a balanced blend of all these elements, forming a foundation for a fulfilling and vibrant life.

Physical wellness is the cornerstone that most people are familiar with. It's about maintaining a healthy body through regular exercise, proper nutrition, and adequate rest. Physical wellness is not merely the absence of disease; it's about functioning at your best and having the energy to meet the demands of daily life. When we take care of our bodies, we set the stage for a healthy and active lifestyle.

Mental wellness, on the other hand, is about nurturing our minds. It involves engaging in activities that stimulate our intellect and creativity, such as reading, solving puzzles, or learning new skills. Mental wellness also encompasses our ability to process information, make decisions, and solve problems. By continuously challenging our minds, we keep them sharp and resilient.

Emotional wellness is all about understanding and managing our emotions. It involves self-awareness, the ability to express and process feelings, and cultivating a positive outlook. Emotional wellness also includes developing coping mechanisms to deal with stress and adversity. By fostering emotional wellness, we create a stable foundation that supports our mental and physical health.

Social wellness focuses on the quality of our relationships and interactions with others. Humans are inherently social creatures, and building meaningful connections with family, friends, and the community is crucial for our well-being. Social wellness involves effective communication, empathy, and the ability to build and maintain healthy relationships. A strong social support network provides emotional security and a sense of belonging.

Spiritual wellness is perhaps the most abstract dimension. It's not necessarily about religion, though for many, it can be. Spiritual wellness is about finding purpose and meaning in life. It involves exploring our values, beliefs, and what gives us a sense of fulfillment. Practices like meditation, reflection, and connecting with nature can enhance our spiritual well-being. By nurturing our spirit, we find a deeper connection to the world and a sense of peace and contentment.

The holistic approach to wellness recognizes that these dimensions are interconnected. A deficiency in one area can impact others. For instance, chronic stress (emotional wellness) can lead to physical health problems, while poor social connections can affect mental health. By striving for balance and harmony among all these aspects, we pave the way for a healthier, more fulfilling life.

The Evolution of Wellness

To truly appreciate the concept of wellness, it's crucial to understand its historical evolution. Wellness is not a modern invention; its roots can be traced back to ancient civilizations. Cultures throughout history have recognized the importance of maintaining balance and harmony within the body and mind, and their approaches to wellness have shaped the practices we know today.

In ancient Greece, wellness was a fundamental part of daily life. The Greeks believed in achieving a balance between the mind, body, and spirit. This holistic approach was epitomized by the famous saying, "a sound mind in a sound body" (Mens sana in corpore sano). Greek physicians like Hippocrates, often referred to as the Father of Medicine, emphasized the importance of diet, exercise, and environmental factors in maintaining health. His teachings laid the groundwork for modern medicine and wellness principles.

Similarly, ancient Eastern philosophies also embraced the concept of holistic wellness. Traditional Chinese Medicine (TCM) and Ayurveda, which originated in India, have been practicing wellness for thousands of years. TCM focuses on achieving harmony between the body's energy (Qi) and its environment through acupuncture, herbal medicine, and Tai Chi. Ayurveda, on the other hand, emphasizes a balanced lifestyle that includes proper nutrition, yoga, and meditation to maintain the equilibrium of the body's doshas (biological energies).

As we move forward in history, the Renaissance period in Europe marked a resurgence of interest in health and wellness. This era saw a renewed focus on the human body, anatomy, and the importance of physical fitness. During this time, artists and scientists began to explore and celebrate the intricacies of the human form, leading to significant advancements in medical knowledge and a greater emphasis on physical well-being.

The 19th and early 20th centuries witnessed the birth of modern public health initiatives, which aimed to address the wellness of entire populations. The industrial revolution brought about rapid urbanization and changes in lifestyle, leading to new health challenges. Public health pioneers like Florence Nightingale revolutionized the approach to healthcare by advocating for sanitation, hygiene, and preventive measures. These efforts helped to establish the foundation for contemporary public health and wellness practices.

In the mid-20th century, the wellness movement began to take shape as we know it today. This period saw the emergence of wellness pioneers like Dr. Halbert Dunn, who coined the term "high-level wellness" in the 1950s. Dunn's work emphasized the importance of personal responsibility and proactive measures in achieving optimal health. The concept of wellness expanded beyond the absence of disease to encompass physical, mental, and emotional well-being.

The 21st century has brought a new wave of wellness awareness, driven by advancements in technology, research, and a growing understanding of the mind-body connection. Today, wellness is a multi-billion-dollar industry, with countless resources available to help individuals lead healthier lives. From fitness apps and wearable technology to wellness retreats and personalized health plans, the tools and knowledge to achieve wellness are more accessible than ever.

Understanding the evolution of wellness helps us appreciate the rich tapestry of knowledge and practices that have shaped our current approach. By learning from the past, we can embrace a more informed and holistic perspective on wellness, one that honors the wisdom of ancient traditions while integrating the latest scientific advancements. As we continue our journey through this book, re-

The Science Behind Wellness

Wellness might seem like a trend driven by popular culture, but it's deeply rooted in science. Understanding the scientific principles behind wellness can help us make informed decisions about our health and adopt practices that are genuinely beneficial. Let's dive into the research that underpins the wellness movement.

First, let's talk about the mind-body connection. Research has shown that our mental state significantly affects our physical health, and vice versa. Chronic stress, for instance, can lead to a host of health problems, including hypertension, heart disease, and a weakened immune system. Conversely, physical activity has been proven to reduce symptoms of depression and anxiety. This bidirectional relationship underscores the importance of addressing both mental and physical health in our wellness journey.

Sleep, often undervalued in our busy lives, plays a critical role in maintaining wellness. Studies have shown that adequate sleep is essential for cognitive function, emotional regulation, and physical health. During sleep, our bodies repair tissues, consolidate memories, and regulate hormones. Chronic sleep deprivation, on the other hand, can lead to a myriad of issues, from impaired judgment and mood swings to increased risk of chronic diseases such as diabetes and obesity. Prioritizing good sleep hygiene is, therefore, a foundational aspect of wellness.

Nutrition science offers compelling evidence on the impact of diet on health. A balanced diet rich in fruits, vegetables, whole grains, and lean proteins can support overall health and prevent chronic diseases. Specific nutrients have been linked to improved mood and cognitive function. For example, omega-3 fatty acids, found in fish and flaxseeds, are known to support brain health and reduce inflammation. The Mediterranean diet, which emphasizes whole foods, healthy fats, and moderate consumption of dairy and meat, has been associated with a lower risk of heart disease and improved longevity.

Physical activity is another cornerstone of wellness supported by extensive research. Regular exercise not only helps in maintaining a healthy weight but also reduces the risk of many chronic diseases, including heart disease, stroke, and certain cancers. Exercise also boosts mental health by releasing endorphins, the body's natural mood lifters, and improving sleep quality. The CDC recommends at least 150 minutes of moderate-intensity aerobic activity or 75 minutes of vigorous-intensity activity each week, combined with muscle-strengthening activities on two or more days per week.

The emerging field of epigenetics provides fascinating insights into how our lifestyle choices can influence our genes. Epigenetics studies how behaviors and environment can cause changes that affect the way our genes work. Unlike genetic changes, epigenetic changes are reversible. For instance, a healthy diet, regular exercise, and stress management can lead to beneficial epigenetic changes, potentially reducing the risk of chronic diseases and improving overall health. This field underscores the power of lifestyle choices in shaping our health outcomes.

Finally, mindfulness and meditation have been extensively studied for their health benefits. Research shows that these practices can reduce stress, improve emotional regulation, and enhance overall well-being. Mindfulness involves staying present and fully engaging with the current moment, which can help reduce the negative impact of stress and increase feelings of calm and happiness. Meditation, on the other hand, involves specific techniques to focus the mind and cultivate a state of relaxed concentration. These practices can rewire the brain, promoting positive changes in areas associated with attention, self-awareness, and emotional regulation.

The science behind wellness provides a robust foundation for our health practices. By understanding the research and evidence supporting various wellness strategies, we can make informed decisions that genuinely enhance our well-being. As we continue to explore the path to wellness, let's keep these scientific insights in mind, using them to guide our choices and actions.

Creating a Personal Wellness Plan

A personal wellness plan is your roadmap to achieving and maintaining optimal health. It is a tailored approach that takes into account your unique needs, goals, and lifestyle. Crafting such a plan involves self-assessment, goal setting, and regular monitoring to ensure that you stay on track and make necessary adjustments along the way.

The first step in creating a personal wellness plan is self-assessment. This involves taking a close look at your current health status and lifestyle. Start by evaluating the various dimensions of wellness: physical, mental, emotional, social, and spiritual. Ask yourself questions like: How often do I exercise? What does my diet look like? How do I handle stress? Am I getting enough sleep? What are my social connections like? Do I engage in activities that fulfill me spiritually? This honest self-reflection will help you identify areas where you are doing well and areas that need improvement.

Once you have a clear understanding of your current state of wellness, it's time to set realistic and specific goals. Your goals should be SMART: Specific, Measurable, Achievable, Relevant, and Time-bound. For example, instead of setting a vague goal like "get fit," aim for something more specific like "exercise for 30 minutes, five days a week." Instead of "eat healthier," try "add three servings of vegetables to my daily diet." Setting clear, achievable goals makes it easier to track your progress and stay motivated.

Next, develop a plan of action to achieve your goals. This plan should include practical steps and strategies tailored to your lifestyle. For instance, if your goal is to exercise regularly, plan out your workouts and schedule them into your calendar. Find activities you enjoy, whether it's jogging, yoga, or dancing, to make it easier to stick to your routine. If you aim to improve your diet, start by making small, manageable changes, like swapping sugary snacks for fruits or incorporating more whole grains into your meals. The key is to make gradual adjustments that you can sustain over time.

Monitoring your progress is crucial for staying on track and making adjustments as needed. Keep a wellness journal or use a health app to track your activities, habits, and how you feel. Regularly review your progress and celebrate your achievements, no matter how small. If you find that certain strategies aren't working, don't be discouraged. Adjust your plan and try new approaches until you find what works best for you. Remember, wellness is a journey, and it's normal to encounter obstacles and setbacks along the way.

Finally, stay committed to your wellness plan by building a support system. Share your goals with friends, family, or a wellness coach who can offer encouragement and accountability. Join wellness groups or online communities to connect with others who share similar goals. Engaging with a supportive network can make your journey more enjoyable and help you stay motivated.

Creating a personal wellness plan empowers you to take control of your health and well-being. It provides a structured framework that guides you towards making positive changes in your life. By setting clear goals, developing actionable steps, and regularly monitoring your progress, you can achieve a balanced and fulfilling state of wellness. Remember, this plan is a living document that evolves as you grow and change. Embrace the journey, stay flexible, and keep moving forward on your path to wellness.

Chapter 2: The Role of Nutrition

Foundations of a Balanced Diet

Summary: Dive into the basics of what constitutes a balanced diet. Discuss macronutrients (proteins, carbohydrates, fats) and micronutrients (vitamins, minerals). Explain their roles in the body and the importance of balance. Provide guidelines on how to create balanced meals and highlight common dietary guidelines.

Nutritional Needs Across Different Life Stages

Summary: Explore how nutritional requirements change from infancy through old age. Discuss specific dietary needs for children, teenagers, adults, and seniors. Include considerations for special populations such as pregnant women and athletes. Highlight the importance of adapting diet to support growth, development, and aging.

Impact of Diet on Physical Health

Summary: Examine the connection between diet and physical health. Discuss how proper nutrition can prevent and manage chronic diseases such as heart disease, diabetes, and obesity. Highlight the role of diet in maintaining a healthy weight, boosting the immune system, and supporting overall bodily functions.

Psychological and Emotional Effects of Nutrition

Summary: Address how diet affects mental and emotional well-being. Discuss the link between nutrition and mood, cognitive function, and mental health conditions like depression and anxiety. Highlight specific nutrients that support brain health and emotional stability. Provide tips on incorporating these nutrients into daily meals.

Practical Strategies for Healthy Eating

Summary: Offer practical advice for incorporating healthy eating habits into daily life. Discuss meal planning, reading food labels, and making healthier choices when eating out. Provide strategies for overcoming common barriers to healthy eating, such as time constraints and budget limitations. Include tips on mindful eating and maintaining long-term dietary changes.

This structure will help lay a comprehensive foundation on the role of nutrition in achieving wellness. Ready to dive into writing any of these points, or something else on your mind?

Embarking on the journey to wellness begins with understanding the bedrock of good health: a balanced diet. The foods we choose to consume play a pivotal role in fueling our bodies, supporting bodily functions, and maintaining overall well-being. At its core, a balanced diet ensures that we receive all the essential nutrients our bodies need to function optimally.

A balanced diet is comprised of macronutrients and micronutrients. Macronutrients, which include proteins, carbohydrates, and fats, are required in larger quantities and provide the energy necessary for daily activities. Proteins are the building blocks of the body, playing a crucial role in the growth, repair, and maintenance of tissues. They are found in foods such as lean meats, poultry, fish, beans, nuts, and dairy products.

Carbohydrates are the body's primary source of energy. They are found in foods like grains, fruits, vegetables, and legumes. It's important to focus on complex carbohydrates, such as whole grains, which provide sustained energy and are rich in fiber, aiding in digestion and preventing spikes in blood sugar levels.

Fats, although often misunderstood, are essential for the absorption of vitamins and the protection of organs. Healthy fats, such as those found in avocados, nuts, seeds, and olive oil, support brain health and provide long-lasting energy. It's important to limit the intake of saturated and trans fats, often found in processed foods, as they can contribute to chronic diseases.

Micronutrients, including vitamins and minerals, are needed in smaller quantities but are equally vital for health. Vitamins such as A, C, D, E, and the B-complex group support various bodily functions, from immune defense to energy production. Minerals like calcium, potassium, and iron are essential for bone health, muscle function, and oxygen transport in the blood. A diet rich in fruits, vegetables, whole grains, and lean proteins typically provides a sufficient amount of these micronutrients.

Creating balanced meals involves combining these nutrients in the right proportions. The "plate method" is a simple and effective way to visualize a balanced meal. Ideally, half of your plate should consist of fruits and vegetables, a quarter should be dedicated to lean proteins, and the remaining quarter should be filled with whole grains. Incorporating a source of healthy fat, such as a drizzle of olive oil or a handful of nuts, rounds out the meal.

Hydration is another crucial aspect of a balanced diet. Water is essential for nearly every bodily function, from regulating temperature to aiding digestion and transporting nutrients. It's important to drink enough water throughout the day, aiming for at least eight

8-ounce glasses, though individual needs may vary based on activity level and climate.

Eating a variety of foods is key to obtaining a wide range of nutrients. Each food group offers unique benefits, and diversity in your diet ensures that you cover all nutritional bases. Additionally, consuming seasonal and locally-sourced produce can enhance nutrient intake and support sustainable practices.

Understanding food labels can also empower you to make healthier choices. Look for labels that highlight essential nutrients and avoid those with excessive amounts of added sugars, sodium, and unhealthy fats. Being mindful of portion sizes and serving recommendations can help prevent overeating and maintain a healthy weight.

In summary, the foundation of a balanced diet lies in the thoughtful combination of macronutrients and micronutrients, adequate hydration, and variety in food choices. By prioritizing whole, unprocessed foods and paying attention to portion sizes, you can create a diet that supports long-term health and well-being. This balanced approach to nutrition sets the stage for the chapters to come, where we will delve deeper into specific dietary needs and practical strategies for healthy eating.

Nutritional Needs Across Different Life Stages

As we journey through different stages of life, our nutritional needs change dramatically. From the rapid growth of infancy to the steady metabolism of old age, each phase requires unique dietary considerations to support development, health, and well-being.

In infancy and childhood, nutrition plays a crucial role in growth and development. During the first year of life, infants require breast milk or formula to provide essential nutrients and antibodies that support immune function. As children grow, their diets should include a variety of foods from all food groups. Protein is vital for muscle development, while carbohydrates provide the energy needed for their active lives. Vitamins and minerals, such as calcium and vitamin D, are necessary for strong bones and teeth. Encouraging healthy eating habits early on helps set the foundation for a lifetime of good nutrition.

As children transition into adolescence, their nutritional needs continue to evolve. This period of rapid growth and hormonal changes requires increased caloric intake and specific nutrients to support development. Protein remains essential for muscle growth, while iron is particularly important for adolescent girls to compensate for menstrual losses. Calcium and vitamin D are critical for bone health, as peak bone mass is typically reached during this stage. Adolescents should be encouraged to make healthy food choices, despite the allure of fast food and sugary snacks, to support their overall health and well-being.

Adulthood brings its own set of nutritional requirements, largely influenced by lifestyle, activity level, and metabolic rate. A balanced diet rich in fruits, vegetables, lean proteins, and whole grains supports energy levels, cognitive function, and disease prevention. Fiber becomes increasingly important in adulthood to aid digestion and reduce the risk of chronic diseases such as heart disease and type 2 diabetes. Healthy fats, particularly omega-3 fatty acids found in fish and flaxseeds, support brain health and reduce inflammation. Adults should also pay attention to portion sizes and make mindful eating choices to maintain a healthy weight.

Pregnancy and breastfeeding introduce additional nutritional considerations. Pregnant women need increased amounts of certain nutrients to support the growing fetus and prepare their bodies for breastfeeding. Folate, iron, and calcium are particularly important during pregnancy. Folate helps prevent neural tube defects, while iron supports increased blood volume and the development of the baby's brain and other organs. Calcium is vital for the development of the baby's bones and teeth. Breastfeeding mothers need extra calories and nutrients to produce milk and maintain their own health. A diet rich in diverse nutrients supports both mother and baby during this critical time.

As we enter older adulthood, our metabolism slows, and our bodies require fewer calories but an increased focus on nutrient density. Protein remains important for maintaining muscle mass and strength, while calcium and vitamin D continue to be essential for bone health. Older adults may also benefit from increased intake of fiber to support digestive health and prevent constipation. Hydration becomes more critical, as the sense of thirst often diminishes with age. Additionally, certain vitamins and minerals, such as vitamin B12 and magnesium, may become more challenging to absorb, necessitating dietary adjustments or supplementation.

Throughout all life stages, it's important to recognize the influence of lifestyle and individual health conditions on nutritional needs. Factors such as physical activity, stress levels, and existing medical conditions can impact dietary requirements. A personalized approach to nutrition, tailored to an individual's specific needs and circumstances, is key to achieving and maintaining optimal health.

By understanding and adapting to the changing nutritional needs across different life stages, we can support our bodies and minds through every phase of life. Nourishing ourselves with the right nutrients at the right times ensures that we not only survive but thrive, enjoying vibrant health and well-being throughout our journey.

Impact of Diet on Physical Health

The connection between diet and physical health is profound and well-documented. What we eat directly influences our body's ability to function, fight disease, and maintain energy levels. A well-balanced diet is a cornerstone of good health, playing a crucial role in preventing and managing various chronic conditions.

Firstly, proper nutrition is essential in maintaining a healthy weight. Obesity is a significant risk factor for numerous health issues, including heart disease, diabetes, and certain cancers. By consuming a balanced diet rich in whole foods—such as fruits, vegetables, whole grains, lean proteins, and healthy fats—we can manage our weight effectively. These foods provide essential nutrients without excessive calories, helping to prevent weight gain and its associated health risks.

Heart health is greatly influenced by diet. Cardiovascular diseases, such as heart disease and stroke, are leading causes of death worldwide. Diets high in saturated fats, trans fats, and cholesterol can contribute to the development of atherosclerosis, a condition where arteries become clogged with fatty deposits. On the other hand, a heart-healthy diet rich in fruits, vegetables, whole grains, and lean proteins can lower the risk of these diseases. Foods high in fiber, such as oats, beans, and whole grains, help reduce cholesterol levels, while omega-3 fatty acids found in fish, flaxseeds, and walnuts support heart health by reducing inflammation and improving blood vessel function.

Diabetes management and prevention are also closely linked to diet. Type 2 diabetes, in particular, is often associated with poor dietary habits and obesity. Consuming a diet high in refined sugars and processed foods can lead to insulin resistance and elevated blood sugar levels. In contrast, a diet that emphasizes complex carbohydrates, fiber, lean proteins, and healthy fats can help regulate blood sugar levels and improve insulin sensitivity. For individuals with diabetes, careful meal planning and portion control are vital to managing the condition and preventing complications.

The immune system relies on a diverse range of nutrients to function effectively. Vitamins and minerals, such as vitamins A, C, D, and E, as well as zinc and selenium, play critical roles in supporting immune function. A diet rich in fruits, vegetables, nuts, and seeds provides these essential nutrients. For example, citrus fruits and leafy greens are excellent sources of vitamin C, which is known for its immune-boosting properties. Additionally, foods like yogurt and kefir contain probiotics that promote a healthy gut microbiome, which is closely linked to immune health.

Bone health is another area where diet plays a pivotal role. Calcium and vitamin D are essential for maintaining strong bones and preventing conditions like osteoporosis. Dairy products, leafy greens, and fortified foods are excellent sources of calcium, while vitamin D can be obtained from sunlight exposure and foods like fatty fish and fortified dairy alternatives. Adequate intake of these nutrients is particularly important during childhood and adolescence when bone development is at its peak, as well as in older adulthood to prevent bone density loss.

Lastly, diet significantly impacts digestive health. A diet high in fiber from fruits, vegetables, whole grains, and legumes promotes regular bowel movements and prevents constipation. Fiber also supports a healthy gut microbiome by providing food for beneficial bacteria. Additionally, staying hydrated and including fermented foods, such as yogurt and sauerkraut, can further enhance digestive health and prevent issues like irritable bowel syndrome (IBS) and inflammatory bowel disease (IBD).

In summary, a well-balanced diet is fundamental to physical health. By making mindful food choices and prioritizing nutrient-dense foods, we can support our body's functions, prevent and manage chronic diseases, and enhance overall well-being. As we continue to explore the role of nutrition, remember that the foods we eat are powerful tools in our journey toward optimal health.

Psychological and Emotional Effects of Nutrition

The food we consume not only fuels our bodies but also significantly impacts our psychological and emotional well-being. Nutrition plays a crucial role in maintaining mental health, influencing mood, cognitive function, and even the development of mental health disorders. Understanding the connection between diet and mental health can help us make informed choices that support overall well-being.

One of the most well-known connections between nutrition and mental health is the impact of diet on mood. Certain nutrients have been shown to affect the production and function of neurotransmitters, the chemicals in the brain that regulate mood and emotions. For example, serotonin, often referred to as the "feel-good" neurotransmitter, is influenced by the availability of tryptophan, an amino acid found in protein-rich foods like turkey, chicken, and legumes. Consuming a diet that includes a variety of protein sources can help maintain healthy levels of serotonin, which in turn supports emotional stability and a positive mood.

Omega-3 fatty acids, primarily found in fatty fish such as salmon, mackerel, and sardines, as well as flaxseeds and walnuts, have been linked to improved mental health. These essential fats play a role in brain function and structure, and research suggests they can help reduce symptoms of depression and anxiety. Omega-3s are believed to exert their effects by reducing inflammation in the brain and promoting the production of anti-inflammatory molecules. Including sources of omega-3 fatty acids in your diet can support mental well-being and cognitive health.

Blood sugar levels also significantly impact mood and energy levels. Consuming refined sugars and simple carbohydrates can lead to rapid spikes and subsequent crashes in blood sugar, which can result in mood swings, irritability, and fatigue. On the other hand, complex carbohydrates, such as whole grains, vegetables, and legumes, provide a steady release of energy, helping to maintain stable blood sugar levels and support consistent mood and energy throughout the day. Incorporating these complex carbohydrates into your diet can help prevent the rollercoaster effect of blood sugar fluctuations.

Vitamins and minerals play a vital role in supporting mental health. B vitamins, particularly B6, B12, and folate, are essential for brain function and the production of neurotransmitters. Deficiencies in these vitamins have been linked to increased risk of depression and cognitive decline. Leafy greens, whole grains, eggs, and fortified cereals are excellent sources of B vitamins. Similarly, minerals like magnesium, zinc, and iron are crucial for brain health. Magnesium, found in nuts, seeds, and dark chocolate, helps regulate the body's stress response, while zinc and iron support cognitive function and mood regulation.

The gut-brain connection is an emerging area of research that highlights the impact of gut health on mental health. The gut microbiome, the community of bacteria living in our digestive tract, plays a significant role in regulating mood and cognitive function. A diet rich in fiber, fermented foods, and probiotics supports a healthy gut microbiome, which in turn can enhance mental well-being. Foods like yogurt, kefir, sauerkraut, and kimchi provide beneficial bacteria that promote gut health. Additionally, prebiotic foods, such as garlic, onions, and bananas, nourish these beneficial bacteria.

Hydration also plays a critical role in mental health. Dehydration can lead to impaired cognitive function, difficulty concentrating, and mood disturbances. Ensuring adequate water intake throughout the day supports brain function and overall well-being.

Incorporating mindful eating practices can further enhance the psychological and emotional benefits of nutrition. Mindful eating involves paying attention to the sensory experience of eating, recognizing hunger and fullness cues, and making conscious food choices. This practice can help foster a healthier relationship with food, reduce emotional eating, and promote overall well-being.

In summary, nutrition has a profound impact on psychological and emotional health. By making mindful, nutrient-rich food choices, we can support brain function, stabilize mood, and enhance overall mental well-being. As we continue exploring the role of nutrition, remember that what we eat affects not only our physical health but also our mind and emotions, shaping our journey toward holistic wellness.

That rounds off the connection between diet and mental health. Shall we move on to the final point, or anything you'd like to revisit?

Practical Strategies for Healthy Eating

Adopting healthy eating habits can seem daunting, especially with the plethora of dietary advice available. However, by integrating practical strategies into your daily routine, you can make healthy eating a manageable and sustainable part of your life. This section will provide actionable tips to help you navigate the journey toward better nutrition.

One of the foundational strategies for healthy eating is meal planning. Planning your meals ahead of time helps ensure that you make nutritious choices and avoid the temptation of unhealthy options.

Start by setting aside time each week to plan your meals and create a grocery list. Focus on incorporating a variety of food groups to ensure a balanced diet. When shopping, stick to your list to avoid impulse buys that may derail your healthy eating goals. Preparing meals in advance, such as cooking in bulk on weekends, can save time during busy weekdays and make it easier to stick to your plan.

Understanding and reading food labels is another essential skill for making healthier choices. Food labels provide valuable information about the nutritional content of packaged foods. Pay attention to serving sizes, as the nutritional information is often based on a specific portion. Look for products that are high in essential nutrients, such as fiber, protein, vitamins, and minerals, and low in added sugars, sodium, and unhealthy fats. Avoid items with long lists of ingredients, especially those with artificial additives and preservatives. By becoming a savvy label reader, you can make more informed decisions about the foods you consume.

Making healthier choices when eating out can be challenging, but with a few strategies, it is entirely achievable. When dining at restaurants, look for menu items that are grilled, baked, steamed, or roasted rather than fried. Opt for dishes that include plenty of vegetables, lean proteins, and whole grains. Don't hesitate to ask for modifications, such as dressing on the side or substituting a side salad for fries. Be mindful of portion sizes, as restaurant servings are often larger than what you would typically eat at home. Consider sharing a meal with a friend or packing half to take home for later.

Overcoming common barriers to healthy eating, such as time constraints and budget limitations, requires creativity and planning. For those with limited time, quick and nutritious meals can be a lifesaver. Keep your pantry stocked with staples like canned beans, whole grains, frozen vegetables, and lean proteins that can be quickly assembled into healthy meals. Batch cooking and freezing portions for later can also be a time-efficient way to ensure you have healthy options on hand. For those on a budget, focus on cost-effective, nutrient-dense foods. Buying seasonal produce, shopping sales, and using store brands can help stretch your food dollars. Remember that healthy eating doesn't have to be expensive; simple, whole foods like eggs, oats, and beans are both affordable and nutritious.

Mindful eating is a practice that can enhance your relationship with food and support healthier choices. Mindful eating involves paying attention to the sensory experience of eating—savoring flavors, textures, and aromas—and recognizing hunger and fullness cues. Avoid distractions like television or smartphones during meals, as they can lead to overeating. Eat slowly and take the time to enjoy your food, which can help you feel more satisfied and less likely to reach for additional servings. Mindful eating also encourages you to listen to your body and make food choices that truly nourish and satisfy you.

Maintaining long-term dietary changes is often the biggest challenge in adopting a healthy eating lifestyle. It's important to approach this journey with flexibility and self-compassion. Allow yourself occasional indulgences without guilt, as strict deprivation can lead to unhealthy relationships with food. Focus on progress rather than perfection, and celebrate small victories along the way. Enlist the support of friends, family, or a health professional to help keep you motivated and accountable. Remember that healthy eating is a lifelong journey, and it's okay to make adjustments as you learn what works best for you.

In summary, adopting practical strategies for healthy eating can make the transition to a nutritious diet both manageable and enjoyable. By planning meals, reading food labels, making mindful choices when dining out, and overcoming common barriers, you can create a sustainable approach to nutrition that supports your overall well-being. Embrace the journey and take pride in each step you take toward a healthier lifestyle.

Chapter 3: Physical Activity and Fitness

The Benefits of Physical Activity

Summary: Discuss the multitude of benefits associated with regular physical activity. Include physical benefits like improved cardiovascular health, stronger muscles and bones, and weight management. Also, cover mental health benefits such as reduced stress, improved mood, and enhanced cognitive function. Highlight the overall impact on longevity and quality of life.

Types of Exercise and Their Benefits

Summary: Explore different types of exercise: aerobic (cardio), strength training, flexibility exercises, and balance training. Describe the unique benefits of each type and how they contribute to overall fitness. Provide examples of activities within each category, such as running, weightlifting, yoga, and Tai Chi.

Creating a Balanced Fitness Routine

Summary: Guide readers on how to create a balanced fitness routine that incorporates various types of exercise. Offer advice on setting realistic fitness goals and designing a weekly schedule that includes cardio, strength, flexibility, and rest days. Discuss the importance of consistency and progressive overload for continuous improvement.

Overcoming Common Barriers to Exercise

Summary: Address common obstacles to regular physical activity, such as lack of time, motivation, and access to facilities. Provide practical solutions to overcome these barriers, including home workouts, time management strategies, and finding activities that are enjoyable. Emphasize the importance of making exercise a habit and integrating it into daily life.

Exercise Safety and Injury Prevention

Summary: Highlight the importance of exercising safely to prevent injuries. Cover essential safety tips, such as proper warm-up and cool-down routines, using correct form and technique, and listening to the body's signals. Discuss common exercise-related injuries and how to avoid them. Provide guidance on seeking professional advice and adapting workouts to individual fitness levels and conditions.

This structure should provide a comprehensive and engaging look at physical activity and fitness, helping readers understand how to incorporate exercise into their lives effectively. Ready to dive into writing any of these points, or something else in mind?

Regular physical activity is a cornerstone of good health, offering a multitude of benefits that extend far beyond the obvious physical improvements. Engaging in consistent exercise can significantly enhance both our physical and mental well-being, contributing to a longer, healthier, and more fulfilling life.

From a physical health perspective, one of the most notable benefits of regular exercise is improved cardiovascular health. Activities such as walking, running, cycling, and swimming elevate heart rate, which strengthens the heart muscle, improves circulation, and boosts overall cardiovascular function. This leads to a reduced risk of heart disease, high blood pressure, stroke, and other cardiovascular conditions. Furthermore, regular physical activity helps maintain a healthy weight by burning calories and building muscle mass, which increases metabolic rate.

Exercise also plays a crucial role in strengthening muscles and bones. Weight-bearing exercises, such as resistance training, weightlifting, and bodyweight exercises, stimulate muscle growth and enhance bone density. This is particularly important for preventing osteoporosis and sarcopenia, conditions characterized by weakened bones and muscle loss, respectively. Stronger muscles and bones contribute to better posture, balance, and overall physical stability, reducing the risk of falls and injuries, especially as we age.

The benefits of physical activity extend to metabolic health as well. Regular exercise improves insulin sensitivity, which helps regulate blood sugar levels and prevent type 2 diabetes. It also lowers levels of LDL (bad) cholesterol and triglycerides while raising levels of HDL (good) cholesterol, contributing to improved lipid profiles and reduced risk of metabolic syndrome. These metabolic improvements collectively reduce the risk of chronic diseases and support overall health.

Beyond the physical benefits, exercise has a profound impact on mental health. Physical activity is known to release endorphins, the body's natural mood elevators. These "feel-good" hormones help reduce stress, anxiety, and symptoms of depression, promoting a more positive and stable emotional state. Regular exercise has also been linked to improved sleep quality, which in turn enhances mental clarity and reduces fatigue.

Cognitive function is another area where exercise makes a significant impact. Studies have shown that physical activity can enhance brain health by promoting neuroplasticity—the brain's ability to adapt and form new neural connections. This leads to improved memory, learning, and cognitive performance. Regular exercise has also been associated with a reduced risk of cognitive decline and neurodegenerative diseases such as Alzheimer's.

In addition to these benefits, physical activity promotes longevity and a better quality of life. Individuals who engage in regular exercise tend to live longer and experience a higher quality of life. They are more likely to maintain their independence, mobility, and functional abilities as they age. The social aspects of physical activity, such as participating in group sports or fitness classes, also contribute to overall well-being by fostering a sense of community and reducing feelings of isolation.

The benefits of physical activity are far-reaching and multifaceted. By incorporating regular exercise into our daily routines, we can enjoy improved cardiovascular health, stronger muscles and bones, better metabolic function, enhanced mental health, and cognitive benefits. Ultimately, the commitment to physical activity is an investment in our long-term health and well-being, paving the way for a more vibrant and fulfilling life.

Types of Exercise and Their Benefits

Understanding the different types of exercise and their unique benefits is essential for creating a well-rounded fitness routine. Each type of exercise offers distinct advantages that contribute to overall physical fitness and health. Let's explore the primary categories of exercise: aerobic (cardio), strength training, flexibility exercises, and balance training.

Aerobic Exercise (Cardio) Aerobic exercise, commonly referred to as cardio, includes activities that increase your heart rate and breathing while working your large muscle groups. Examples of aerobic exercise include walking, running, cycling, swimming, and dancing. The benefits of cardio are extensive and well-documented.

Regular aerobic exercise improves cardiovascular health by strengthening the heart and enhancing blood circulation. This helps lower the risk of heart disease, high blood pressure, and stroke. Additionally, cardio exercises increase lung capacity and endurance, making daily activities easier and less tiring. Cardio is also effective for weight management, as it burns calories and boosts metabolism. Moreover, aerobic exercise has significant mental health benefits, such as reducing stress, anxiety, and symptoms of depression, while enhancing mood and cognitive function.

Strength Training Strength training, also known as resistance or weight training, involves exercises that improve muscular strength and endurance. This type of exercise can be performed using free weights, weight machines, resistance bands, or bodyweight exercises like push-ups and squats. The primary benefit of strength training is the development of stronger muscles and increased muscle mass. Building muscle not only enhances physical strength but also supports metabolic health by increasing the body's resting metabolic rate, which helps with weight management. Strength training improves bone density, reducing the risk of osteoporosis and fractures. Additionally, it enhances joint stability, balance, and coordination, which are crucial for preventing injuries and maintaining mobility, especially as we age. Strength training also contributes to better posture and can alleviate chronic conditions such as back pain.

Flexibility Exercises Flexibility exercises aim to enhance the range of motion of your muscles and joints. Activities like stretching, yoga, and Pilates are common forms of flexibility training. The benefits of flexibility exercises include improved muscle elasticity and joint mobility, which help prevent injuries and reduce muscle soreness. Enhanced flexibility can lead to better posture, greater ease of movement, and reduced risk of muscle strains. Flexibility exercises are particularly beneficial for reducing tension and stress, as they promote relaxation and a sense of well-being. Practicing yoga, for example, combines flexibility with mindfulness and breathing techniques, offering both physical and mental health benefits. Regular stretching can also alleviate stiffness and pain associated with sedentary lifestyles or repetitive motions.

Balance Training Balance training focuses on improving stability and coordination. It involves exercises that challenge your balance, such as standing on one leg, using balance boards, or practicing Tai Chi. Balance training is essential for enhancing proprioception, which is your body's ability to sense its position and movement in space. Improved balance helps prevent falls and injuries, particularly in older adults. It also supports better coordination and agility, which are important for performing everyday activities and sports. Balance training can enhance athletic performance and improve core strength, leading to greater overall stability and posture.

Incorporating a variety of these exercises into your fitness routine ensures a comprehensive approach to health and wellness. Aerobic exercise improves cardiovascular and respiratory health, strength training builds muscle and bone density, flexibility exercises enhance range of motion and reduce tension, and balance training promotes stability and coordination. By understanding the benefits of each type of exercise, you can create a balanced fitness plan that supports your overall well-being and helps you achieve your health goals.

Creating a Balanced Fitness Routine

Designing a balanced fitness routine is essential for achieving your health goals and maintaining overall wellness. A well-rounded exercise plan incorporates various types of workouts, ensuring that you address all aspects of fitness, from cardiovascular health to muscular strength, flexibility, and balance. Here's how to create a comprehensive fitness routine that keeps you motivated and consistently progressing.

Setting Realistic Fitness Goals The first step in creating a balanced fitness routine is setting clear, realistic goals. Consider what you want to achieve through your fitness plan—whether it's improving cardiovascular health, building muscle, increasing flexibility, or maintaining a healthy weight. Setting SMART goals (Specific, Measurable, Achievable, Relevant, and Time-bound) can provide direction and motivation. For example, instead of a vague goal like "get fit," aim for "complete a 5K run in three months" or "perform 10 pull-ups within six weeks." Having concrete goals helps you track progress and stay focused.

Incorporating Different Types of Exercise A balanced fitness routine should include a variety of exercise types to ensure comprehensive fitness development:

Cardio: Aim for at least 150 minutes of moderate-intensity aerobic exercise or 75 minutes of vigorous-intensity aerobic exercise per week, as recommended by the CDC. Activities like brisk walking, running, cycling, swimming, or group fitness classes can improve cardiovascular health and endurance.

Strength Training: Incorporate strength training exercises at least two days a week to build and maintain muscle mass. Use free weights, resistance bands, weight machines, or bodyweight exercises like squats, push-ups, and lunges. Focus on all major muscle groups for balanced muscle development.

Flexibility: Include flexibility exercises, such as stretching, yoga, or Pilates, several times a week to enhance your range of motion and prevent injuries. Flexibility training helps keep your muscles and joints supple and reduces muscle tightness and soreness.

Balance: Add balance training exercises to your routine at least two to three times a week. Activities like Tai Chi, balance board exercises, or simply practicing standing on one leg can improve stability and coordination, which are essential for overall physical fitness and injury prevention.

Designing Your Weekly Schedule To create a balanced fitness routine, distribute these different types of exercises throughout the week. Here's an example of a weekly workout schedule:

Monday: 30 minutes of cardio (e.g., running) + 20 minutes of strength training (upper body)

Tuesday: 20 minutes of flexibility exercises (e.g., yoga) + balance training

Wednesday: 30 minutes of cardio (e.g., cycling)

Thursday: 20 minutes of strength training (lower body) + 20 minutes of flexibility exercises

Friday: 30 minutes of cardio (e.g., swimming)

Saturday: 20 minutes of strength training (full body) + balance training

Sunday: Rest or light activities like walking or stretching

Consistency and Progressive Overload Consistency is key to seeing results from your fitness routine. Commit to your schedule and make exercise a non-negotiable part of your daily life. Additionally, applying the principle of progressive overload—gradually increasing the intensity, duration, or frequency of your workouts—will help you continue to improve and avoid plateaus. For example, increase the weights you lift, add extra repetitions or sets, or incorporate more challenging variations of exercises over time.

Listening to Your Body and Rest Days While it's important to challenge yourself, it's equally crucial to listen to your body and allow for adequate rest and recovery. Overtraining can lead to injuries and burnout, so make sure to schedule rest days or engage in light activities like walking or gentle stretching on those days. Paying attention to your body's signals and giving yourself time to recover ensures long-term success and sustainability in your fitness journey.

By setting realistic goals, incorporating a variety of exercise types, designing a balanced weekly schedule, and maintaining consistency, you can create a fitness routine that supports all aspects of your health and wellness. Remember, the journey to fitness is a marathon, not a sprint. Stay patient, stay committed, and enjoy the process of becoming a healthier, stronger version of yourself.

Overcoming Common Barriers to Exercise

Embarking on a fitness journey is an admirable goal, but many people encounter obstacles that can make regular exercise challenging. Identifying and overcoming these barriers is crucial to maintaining a consistent fitness routine. Whether it's a lack of time, motivation, or access to facilities, there are practical solutions to help you stay active and committed to your health goals.

Lack of Time One of the most common barriers to regular exercise is the perception of having no time. Busy work schedules, family obligations, and other responsibilities can make it seem impossible to fit in a workout. However, integrating exercise into your daily routine is more manageable than it might appear. Start by identifying small pockets of time throughout your day where you can squeeze in physical activity. For instance, a 10-minute walk during lunch breaks, a quick home workout in the morning, or a brief yoga session before bed can accumulate to meet your fitness goals. High-intensity interval training (HIIT) is also an effective option, as it provides a vigorous workout in a short amount of time. Additionally, consider multitasking, such as doing squats or lunges while watching TV or taking the stairs instead of the elevator.

Lack of Motivation Staying motivated can be challenging, especially when the initial excitement of starting a new fitness routine fades. To keep your motivation high, find activities that you genuinely enjoy. Whether it's dancing, hiking, swimming, or playing a sport, engaging in exercises that bring you joy makes it easier to stay committed. Setting short-term and long-term goals can also provide a sense of direction and achievement. Keep a workout journal to track your progress and celebrate milestones, no matter how small. Additionally, finding a workout buddy or joining a fitness group can offer accountability and social support, making exercise more enjoyable and motivating. Remind yourself of the benefits of exercise, such as improved energy levels, better mood, and enhanced overall health, to stay inspired.

Access to Facilities Limited access to fitness facilities or equipment can be a significant barrier, but it doesn't have to halt your progress. Home workouts are a convenient and cost-effective solution that can be just as effective as gym sessions. Utilize bodyweight exercises, such as push-ups, squats, planks, and burpees, which require no equipment and can be done anywhere. Online workout videos and fitness apps offer guided sessions that cater to various fitness levels and preferences. If you prefer equipment, consider investing in a few versatile pieces, such as resistance bands, dumbbells, or a yoga mat. Outdoor activities like walking, running, cycling, or participating in community sports are also great ways to stay active without the need for a gym.

Physical Barriers and Injuries Physical barriers, such as chronic conditions or injuries, can make exercising challenging. It's essential to consult with a healthcare professional before starting or modifying an exercise routine to ensure it's safe for your specific condition. Low-impact exercises, such as swimming, cycling, or yoga, are gentle on the joints and can be effective for individuals with physical limitations. Adaptive fitness programs and specialized equipment are available for those with mobility issues, making exercise more accessible. Gradually increasing the intensity and duration of your workouts can help prevent injury and allow your body to adjust safely to new activities.

Lack of Knowledge A lack of knowledge about how to exercise effectively can be a deterrent. Education is key to overcoming this barrier. Research different types of exercises and their benefits to find what suits your goals and preferences. Many online resources, including videos, articles, and apps, provide detailed instructions and demonstrations for various workouts. Hiring a personal trainer, even temporarily, can offer personalized guidance and help you build confidence in your fitness routine. Fitness classes, whether in-person or virtual, provide structure and instruction, making it easier to learn new exercises and techniques.

In summary, overcoming common barriers to exercise requires creativity, planning, and determination. By addressing these obstacles with practical solutions, you can build a consistent and enjoyable fitness routine that supports your health and well-being. Remember, the key to success is finding what works best for you and staying adaptable in your approach. Keep moving forward, and the benefits of regular exercise will become an integral part of your lifestyle.

Exercise Safety and Injury Prevention

While engaging in regular physical activity is crucial for maintaining health, it's equally important to exercise safely to prevent injuries and maximize the benefits of your workouts. Understanding proper techniques, listening to your body, and implementing injury prevention strategies can help you enjoy a long-term, injury-free fitness journey.

Proper Warm-Up and Cool-Down Routines Warming up before exercise prepares your body for the demands of physical activity by gradually increasing your heart rate and loosening your muscles and joints. A proper warm-up should last 5-10 minutes and include dynamic stretches and light aerobic activities, such as brisk walking or jogging. Dynamic stretches, like leg swings and arm circles, help improve your range of motion and reduce the risk of muscle strains.

Similarly, cooling down after a workout is essential for gradually bringing your heart rate back to its resting state and preventing muscle stiffness. A cool-down should also last 5-10 minutes and include static stretches, such as hamstring stretches or calf stretches, which help improve flexibility and promote muscle recovery. Cooling down with light aerobic activity, like slow walking, can aid in reducing post-exercise muscle soreness and stiffness.

Using Correct Form and Technique Using proper form and technique during exercise is vital for preventing injuries and ensuring that you get the most out of your workouts. Incorrect form can place unnecessary stress on your muscles, joints, and ligaments, leading to strains, sprains, and overuse injuries. It's essential to learn the correct techniques for each exercise, whether you're lifting weights, running, or practicing yoga.

If you're unsure about your form, consider seeking guidance from a certified fitness professional or using instructional videos from reputable sources. Focus on performing each movement with control and alignment, paying attention to your body mechanics. For example, when performing a squat, ensure that your knees do not extend past your toes, and keep your back straight to avoid placing excessive strain on your lower back.

Listening to Your Body Listening to your body is crucial for preventing injuries and ensuring a sustainable fitness routine. Pay attention to any signs of discomfort or pain during exercise, and do not ignore them. Pain is your body's way of signaling that something is wrong, and continuing to push through it can lead to more serious injuries. If you experience sharp or persistent pain, stop the activity immediately and seek medical advice if necessary.

It's also important to recognize the difference between normal exercise-related soreness and pain that indicates injury. Mild muscle soreness, known as delayed onset muscle soreness (DOMS), is common after a workout, especially if you are trying new exercises or increasing intensity. However, if you experience severe pain, swelling, or a decrease in range of motion, it may indicate an injury that requires attention.

Preventing Overuse Injuries Overuse injuries occur when repetitive stress is placed on a particular part of the body without adequate rest and recovery. Common overuse injuries include shin splints, tendonitis, and stress fractures. To prevent overuse injuries, incorporate variety into your workouts by cross-training and alternating different types of exercises. For example, combine running with swimming or cycling to reduce the repetitive impact on your joints.

Adequate rest and recovery are also essential for preventing overuse injuries. Allow your body time to recover between intense workouts by scheduling rest days or engaging in low-impact activities like stretching or walking. Ensure that you get enough sleep, as it plays a critical role in muscle repair and recovery.

Seeking Professional Advice If you are new to exercise or have specific health concerns, seeking professional advice can help you exercise safely and effectively. A certified personal trainer can create a customized fitness plan that aligns with your goals and fitness level while teaching you proper techniques. Additionally, if you have any pre-existing medical conditions or injuries, consult with a healthcare provider before starting a new exercise program to ensure that it is safe for you.

In summary, exercising safely is crucial for preventing injuries and maintaining a long-term fitness routine. By incorporating proper warm-up and cool-down routines, using correct form and technique, listening to your body, preventing overuse injuries, and seeking professional advice when needed, you can enjoy the benefits of physical activity while minimizing the risk of injury. Remember, your safety and well-being should always come first in your fitness journey.

Chapter 4: Mental Health Matters

Understanding Mental Health

Summary: Define what mental health encompasses, including emotional, psychological, and social well-being. Discuss the stigma surrounding mental health and the importance of addressing it. Highlight how mental health affects our thoughts, feelings, and behaviors and why it's a crucial part of overall health.

Common Mental Health Issues

Summary: Explore common mental health disorders such as anxiety, depression, bipolar disorder, and PTSD. Explain the symptoms, causes, and potential impacts on daily life. Discuss the importance of early detection and seeking professional help.

Stress Management and Coping Mechanisms

Summary: Discuss the different types of stress and their effects on mental health. Provide strategies for managing stress, including relaxation techniques, time management, and healthy lifestyle choices. Introduce the concept of resilience and how to build it.

The Role of Therapy and Counseling

Summary: Explain the various types of therapy and counseling available, such as cognitive-behavioral therapy (CBT), psychotherapy, and counseling. Discuss how these treatments can help individuals manage their mental health, overcome challenges, and improve quality of life. Highlight the benefits of seeking professional support.

Self-Care and Mental Well-Being

Summary: Emphasize the importance of self-care practices in maintaining mental health. Provide practical tips for daily self-care routines, including mindfulness, exercise, healthy eating, and social connections. Discuss the role of hobbies and leisure activities in mental well-being.

This outline will provide a comprehensive understanding of mental health and offer practical advice to support and maintain mental well-being. Ready to dive into writing any of these points, or something else in mind?

Mental health is a vital component of our overall well-being, yet it is often misunderstood and surrounded by stigma. At its core, mental health encompasses our emotional, psychological, and social well-being. It influences how we think, feel, and act, shaping our ability to handle stress, relate to others, and make decisions. Understanding mental health is crucial for fostering a balanced and fulfilling life.

Emotional well-being involves the capacity to manage and express emotions appropriately. It's about experiencing a full range of emotions, from happiness and contentment to sadness and anger, in ways that are constructive and not overwhelming. Emotional well-being allows us to navigate life's ups and downs with resilience, maintaining a sense of balance even during challenging times.

Psychological well-being relates to our cognitive processes, such as thinking, learning, and memory. It involves having a positive outlook on life, maintaining self-esteem, and feeling a sense of purpose and achievement. Psychological well-being is nurtured by engaging in activities that stimulate the mind, fostering creativity, and pursuing goals that align with our values and interests.

Social well-being refers to our ability to form and maintain healthy relationships. It's about feeling connected to others, having a support network, and effectively communicating and interacting with those around us. Social well-being is enhanced by building meaningful connections, participating in community activities, and cultivating empathy and understanding.

Mental health is not static; it fluctuates throughout our lives based on various factors, including life experiences, biological predispositions, and environmental influences. Just as physical health can vary, so too can mental health, and it's essential to recognize that everyone experiences periods of mental well-being and distress.

Unfortunately, stigma surrounding mental health persists, often preventing individuals from seeking the help they need. Misconceptions and negative attitudes about mental health conditions can lead to feelings of shame and isolation. Challenging these stigmas and promoting open conversations about mental health is vital for creating a supportive and inclusive society where individuals feel empowered to seek help without fear of judgment.

The impacts of mental health on our daily lives are profound. Poor mental health can affect every aspect of our lives, from our physical health and relationships to our ability to work and enjoy leisure activities. It can manifest in various ways, such as persistent sadness, anxiety, irritability, or difficulty concentrating. Understanding and addressing mental health is essential for maintaining overall well-being and functioning.

Recognizing the importance of mental health is the first step towards fostering a healthier, more balanced life. By prioritizing mental health, we can improve our emotional resilience, enhance our cognitive abilities, and build stronger social connections. It involves taking proactive steps to maintain mental well-being, such as practicing self-care, seeking therapy, and building a supportive environment.

Addressing mental health is not just about managing disorders; it's about promoting overall wellness and preventing issues before they escalate. This includes recognizing early signs of mental health challenges and taking steps to address them. It's also about understanding that seeking help is a sign of strength, not weakness. Professional support, whether through therapy, counseling, or medication, can provide invaluable tools and strategies for managing mental health.

In conclusion, understanding mental health is fundamental to our overall well-being. It encompasses our emotional, psychological, and social aspects, influencing every part of our lives. By challenging stigma, promoting open conversations, and prioritizing mental health, we can create a more supportive and inclusive environment that fosters well-being for all. Recognize the importance of mental health in your life, and take proactive steps to nurture and maintain it for a balanced and fulfilling existence.

Common Mental Health Issues

Mental health disorders are increasingly recognized as critical public health issues, affecting millions of people worldwide. Understanding common mental health conditions, their symptoms, and their impacts on daily life is essential for raising awareness, reducing stigma, and encouraging early intervention and treatment.

Anxiety Disorders Anxiety disorders are among the most prevalent mental health conditions, characterized by excessive fear, worry, or nervousness. These disorders can manifest in various forms, including generalized anxiety disorder (GAD), panic disorder, social anxiety disorder, and specific phobias. Symptoms of anxiety disorders may include persistent worry, restlessness, fatigue, difficulty concentrating, and physical symptoms such as increased heart rate, sweating, and muscle tension. The causes of anxiety disorders are multifaceted, involving genetic, environmental, and psychological factors. Left untreated, anxiety disorders can significantly impair daily functioning and quality of life. Early detection and treatment through therapy, medication, or a combination of both can help individuals manage their symptoms and lead fulfilling lives.

Depression: Depression, or major depressive disorder (MDD), is a common and serious mental health condition characterized by persistent feelings of sadness, hopelessness, and a lack of interest or pleasure in activities once enjoyed. Other symptoms include changes in appetite and sleep patterns, fatigue, difficulty concentrating, and thoughts of death or suicide. The exact causes of depression are complex and can include genetic predisposition, biochemical imbalances, and stressful life events. Depression affects individuals differently, but it often leads to significant impairments in social, occupational, and daily functioning. Treatment for depression typically involves a combination of psychotherapy, medication, and lifestyle changes. Early intervention is crucial for improving outcomes and helping individuals regain control over their lives.

Bipolar Disorder Bipolar disorder, previously known as manic-depressive illness, is characterized by extreme mood swings, including periods of mania or hypomania (elevated mood and energy levels) and episodes of depression. During manic episodes, individuals may experience heightened energy, reduced need for sleep, grandiosity, impulsive behavior, and rapid speech. Depressive episodes involve symptoms similar to those of major depression. The exact cause of bipolar disorder is not fully understood, but it is believed to involve a combination of genetic, biological, and environmental factors. Bipolar disorder can significantly impact relationships, work, and overall functioning. Effective management typically requires a comprehensive treatment plan that includes medication, psychotherapy, and lifestyle adjustments.

Post-Traumatic Stress Disorder (PTSD) PTSD is a mental health condition triggered by experiencing or witnessing a traumatic event, such as combat, natural disasters, accidents, or assault. Symptoms of PTSD can include intrusive thoughts or memories of the trauma, flashbacks, nightmares, severe anxiety, and avoidance of reminders of the traumatic event. Individuals with PTSD may also experience changes in mood and cognition, such as feelings of detachment, negative beliefs about oneself or others, and difficulty experiencing positive emotions. PTSD can have a profound impact on daily life, affecting relationships, work, and overall well-being. Treatment often involves trauma-focused therapies, such as cognitive-behavioral therapy (CBT) and eye movement desensitization and reprocessing (EMDR), along with medication to manage symptoms.

Obsessive-Compulsive Disorder (OCD) OCD is characterized by persistent, intrusive thoughts (obsessions) and repetitive behaviors or mental acts (compulsions) performed to alleviate the distress caused by the obsessions. Common obsessions include fears of contamination, doubts about safety, and intrusive thoughts about harm. Compulsions may involve behaviors such as excessive cleaning, checking, counting, or seeking reassurance. The exact cause of OCD is not fully understood but may involve genetic, neurological, and environmental factors. OCD can interfere with daily activities and cause significant distress. Treatment typically includes cognitive-behavioral therapy (CBT), particularly exposure and response prevention (ERP), and medication to help manage symptoms.

Understanding these common mental health issues is vital for recognizing the signs and encouraging individuals to seek help. Mental health conditions are treatable, and early intervention can lead to better outcomes. By raising awareness and promoting access to mental health resources, we can create a more supportive and inclusive environment for those affected by these conditions.

Stress Management and Coping Mechanisms

Stress is a ubiquitous part of modern life, impacting mental health significantly. Understanding the different types of stress and learning effective coping mechanisms can greatly enhance our ability to manage it, leading to improved overall well-being.

Types of Stress Stress can be categorized into acute, episodic acute, and chronic stress. Acute stress is the immediate reaction to a new and challenging situation, such as a deadline at work or a sudden change in plans. It is short-term and often resolved quickly. Episodic acute stress occurs when someone frequently experiences acute stress. This might be the case for individuals who constantly face high-pressure situations or have a chaotic lifestyle. Chronic stress, on the other hand, is long-term and can be more damaging. It arises from persistent problems, such as a toxic work environment, ongoing financial issues, or chronic illness. Understanding these different types of stress helps us identify their sources and tailor our coping strategies accordingly.

Effects of Stress on Mental Health Chronic stress can have profound effects on mental health. It can lead to conditions such as anxiety, depression, and burnout. Physically, it can manifest through symptoms like headaches, gastrointestinal issues, and sleep disturbances. Stress activates the body's fight-or-flight response, releasing hormones such as cortisol and adrenaline. While this response is helpful in short bursts, chronic activation can wear the body down, leading to a variety of health problems. Recognizing the signs of stress early and taking proactive steps to manage it is crucial for maintaining mental and physical health.

Relaxation Techniques Relaxation techniques are effective tools for managing stress. Deep breathing exercises, for instance, can help calm the nervous system. Techniques like diaphragmatic breathing involve taking slow, deep breaths, which can lower heart rate and reduce the stress response. Progressive muscle relaxation, which involves tensing and then slowly releasing different muscle groups, can also be beneficial. Another popular method is mindfulness meditation, which encourages focusing on the present moment without judgment. Practicing mindfulness can help reduce anxiety and promote a sense of calm.

Time Management Effective time management can significantly reduce stress levels. Prioritizing tasks, setting realistic goals, and breaking tasks into smaller, manageable steps can prevent feelings of overwhelm. Using tools like planners or digital calendars can help keep track of commitments and deadlines. It's also important to allocate time for breaks and self-care activities to recharge. Learning to say no to additional responsibilities when your plate is already full is a critical skill in managing stress and maintaining balance.

Healthy Lifestyle Choices Maintaining a healthy lifestyle is foundational to stress management. Regular physical activity, such as walking, running, or yoga, helps release endorphins, the body's natural stress relievers. A balanced diet rich in nutrients can also support mental health by stabilizing mood and energy levels. Adequate sleep is essential, as sleep deprivation can exacerbate stress and impair cognitive function. Limiting caffeine and alcohol intake, which can heighten anxiety and disrupt sleep, is also beneficial.

Building Resilience: Resilience is the ability to bounce back from adversity and cope with stress more effectively. Building resilience involves developing a positive mindset, cultivating supportive relationships, and learning from experiences. Practicing gratitude, keeping a journal, and setting aside time for hobbies and activities that bring joy can enhance resilience. Additionally, seeking support from friends, family, or mental health professionals when needed is crucial. Resilience is not about avoiding stress but rather about developing the strength to navigate it successfully.

In summary, stress is an inevitable part of life, but its impact on mental health can be managed through effective coping mechanisms. By understanding the types of stress, practicing relaxation techniques, managing time efficiently, making healthy lifestyle choices, and building resilience, we can improve our ability to handle stress and enhance our overall well-being. Remember, managing stress is an ongoing process that requires regular attention and effort. Embrace these strategies to cultivate a more balanced and fulfilling life.

The Role of Therapy and Counseling

Therapy and counseling play a vital role in managing mental health and improving overall well-being. These therapeutic interventions offer individuals a safe and supportive space to explore their thoughts, emotions, and behaviors, helping them navigate life's challenges and develop coping strategies. Understanding the various types of therapy and their benefits can help individuals make informed decisions about seeking professional support.

Cognitive-Behavioral Therapy (CBT) Cognitive-Behavioral Therapy (CBT) is one of the most widely used and effective forms of therapy for treating a range of mental health conditions, including anxiety, depression, and PTSD. CBT focuses on identifying and challenging negative thought patterns and beliefs that contribute to emotional distress. By learning to recognize and reframe these cognitive distortions, individuals can develop healthier ways of thinking and responding to situations. CBT is structured, goal-oriented, and typically short-term, making it a practical approach for those seeking to address specific issues. The skills learned in CBT can be applied in everyday life, empowering individuals to manage their mental health independently.

Psychotherapy: Psychotherapy, often referred to as talk therapy, encompasses a broad range of therapeutic approaches aimed at helping individuals understand and work through their emotions, thoughts, and behaviors. Unlike CBT, which is more structured, psychotherapy can be open-ended and exploratory, allowing individuals to delve into their past experiences, relationships, and patterns of behavior. Psychotherapy can help individuals gain insight into the underlying causes of their mental health issues, fostering self-awareness and personal growth. It is particularly beneficial for those dealing with complex or long-standing issues, such as trauma, grief, or identity struggles. Psychotherapy can be conducted in individual, group, or family settings, depending on the needs of the individual.

Counseling: Counseling is a therapeutic approach that focuses on providing support and guidance to individuals facing specific life challenges or transitions, such as relationship issues, career changes, or coping with loss. Counselors work with clients to explore their feelings, set goals, and develop action plans to address their concerns. Counseling is typically shorter-term and more focused than psychotherapy, with an emphasis on practical problem-solving and emotional support. It can be a valuable resource for individuals seeking help with immediate or situational issues.

Benefits of Professional Support Seeking professional support through therapy or counseling offers numerous benefits for mental health and overall well-being. One of the primary advantages is having a safe and confidential space to express emotions and thoughts without judgment. Therapists and counselors provide empathy, validation, and a non-biased perspective, helping individuals feel heard and understood.

Therapy and counseling also equip individuals with coping strategies and tools to manage stress, anxiety, depression, and other mental health challenges. These interventions can improve emotional regulation, enhance communication skills, and foster healthier relationships. Additionally, therapy can promote self-discovery and personal growth, empowering individuals to make positive changes in their lives.

Choosing the Right Therapist or Counselor Finding the right therapist or counselor is crucial for a successful therapeutic experience. It's important to consider factors such as the therapist's qualifications, experience, and therapeutic approach. Building a strong rapport and feeling comfortable with the therapist are essential for effective therapy. Many therapists offer initial consultations to help individuals determine if they are a good fit. It's also important to consider logistical factors, such as location, availability, and cost, when choosing a therapist.

Overcoming Barriers to Seeking Help Despite the benefits of therapy and counseling, many individuals hesitate to seek help due to stigma, fear, or uncertainty. Overcoming these barriers involves recognizing that seeking help is a sign of strength and self-care. It's important to educate oneself about the positive impact of therapy and to reach out to trusted individuals for support in making the decision. Online therapy platforms and telehealth services have also made accessing mental health support more convenient and accessible.

In conclusion, therapy and counseling are valuable tools for managing mental health and fostering personal growth. By understanding the different types of therapy and their benefits, individuals can make informed decisions about seeking professional support. Embracing therapy as a proactive step toward well-being can lead to significant improvements in mental health and overall quality of life.

Self-Care and Mental Well-Being

Self-care is a crucial aspect of maintaining mental health and overall well-being. It involves taking intentional actions to care for your physical, emotional, and mental health. Incorporating self-care practices into your daily routine can help you manage stress, enhance your mood, and improve your quality of life. Here's how to integrate self-care into your life effectively.

Mindfulness and Meditation Mindfulness and meditation are powerful tools for managing stress and promoting mental well-being. Mindfulness involves paying attention to the present moment without judgment, allowing you to become more aware of your thoughts, feelings, and sensations. Regular mindfulness practice can help reduce anxiety, improve focus, and enhance emotional regulation. Simple techniques, such as mindful breathing, body scans, and mindful eating, can be easily incorporated into daily routines.

Meditation, a practice that involves focusing the mind and eliminating distractions, can lead to profound mental and emotional benefits. Techniques like guided meditation, loving-kindness meditation, and transcendental meditation can help cultivate a sense of peace and relaxation. Setting aside just a few minutes each day for meditation can significantly impact your mental health, promoting a calmer and more centered state of mind.

Physical Activity Regular physical activity is not only beneficial for physical health but also plays a vital role in mental well-being. Exercise releases endorphins, the body's natural mood elevators, which can help reduce stress and enhance feelings of happiness. Activities like walking, running, yoga, and dancing can be both enjoyable and effective in improving mental health. Finding an activity that you love and making it a regular part of your routine can provide a consistent outlet for stress relief and emotional balance.

Healthy Eating Nutrition has a significant impact on mental health. A balanced diet rich in essential nutrients supports brain function and emotional stability. Foods high in omega-3 fatty acids, such as fish and flaxseeds, have been linked to improved mood and cognitive function. Similarly, fruits, vegetables, whole grains, and lean proteins provide the necessary vitamins and minerals that support mental well-being. Avoiding excessive consumption of caffeine, sugar, and processed foods can also help maintain stable energy levels and prevent mood swings.

Social Connections Human beings are inherently social creatures, and maintaining healthy social connections is crucial for mental health. Strong relationships provide emotional support, reduce feelings of isolation, and enhance overall well-being. Make time to connect with friends, family, and loved ones regularly. Whether through face-to-face interactions, phone calls, or virtual meetings, nurturing your social network can provide a sense of belonging and support during challenging times.

Engaging in Hobbies and Leisure Activities Engaging in hobbies and leisure activities that bring you joy and fulfillment is an essential component of self-care. Pursuing interests outside of work and daily responsibilities can help reduce stress and increase life satisfaction. Whether it's painting, gardening, reading, playing an instrument, or cooking, finding time for activities that you love can provide a valuable outlet for self-expression and relaxation.

Setting Boundaries Setting healthy boundaries is a critical aspect of self-care. Boundaries help protect your mental and emotional energy by defining what is acceptable and what is not in your interactions and relationships. Learn to say no to commitments that overwhelm you and prioritize activities that align with your well-being. Setting boundaries also involves creating a balance between work, personal time, and rest, ensuring that you have time to recharge and care for yourself.

Sleep Hygiene Adequate sleep is fundamental to mental health. Sleep allows the brain to rest, repair, and process emotions, contributing to overall well-being. Practicing good sleep hygiene involves creating a consistent sleep schedule, establishing a relaxing bedtime routine, and creating a sleep-conducive environment. Avoiding stimulants like caffeine and electronic devices before bed can also promote better sleep quality. Prioritizing sleep is essential for maintaining mental clarity, emotional stability, and physical health.

Professional Support While self-care practices are beneficial, there may be times when professional support is necessary. Seeking help from a therapist, counselor, or mental health professional can provide additional tools and strategies for managing mental health challenges. Professional support can offer a safe space to explore deeper issues and develop personalized coping mechanisms.

In conclusion, self-care is a vital practice for maintaining mental health and overall well-being. By incorporating mindfulness, physical activity, healthy eating, social connections, hobbies, boundaries, sleep hygiene, and seeking professional support when needed, you can create a balanced and fulfilling life. Embrace self-care as a continuous, intentional practice that nurtures your mind, body, and spirit, paving the way for lasting mental well-being.

Chapter 5: The Power of Sleep

The Science of Sleep

Summary: Explore the biological processes that occur during sleep. Discuss the stages of sleep, including REM and non-REM sleep, and their significance for physical and mental health. Explain the role of the circadian rhythm in regulating sleep patterns and how it affects overall well-being.

Sleep and Physical Health

Summary: Examine the impact of sleep on physical health. Discuss how adequate sleep contributes to bodily functions such as immune system support, hormone regulation, and cellular repair. Highlight the consequences of sleep deprivation on physical health, including increased risk of chronic conditions like heart disease, diabetes, and obesity.

Sleep and Mental Health

Summary: Investigate the connection between sleep and mental health. Explain how sleep affects cognitive functions, mood regulation, and emotional resilience. Discuss the bidirectional relationship between sleep disorders and mental health conditions, such as anxiety and depression, and the importance of addressing sleep issues to support mental well-being.

Common Sleep Disorders and Their Management

Summary: Identify common sleep disorders, such as insomnia, sleep apnea, restless legs syndrome, and narcolepsy. Provide an overview of their symptoms, causes, and impacts on daily life. Offer practical advice for managing and treating these disorders, including lifestyle changes, medical interventions, and therapeutic approaches.

Strategies for Improving Sleep Quality

Summary: Offer practical tips and strategies for enhancing sleep quality. Discuss the importance of establishing a regular sleep routine, creating a sleep-conducive environment, and adopting healthy sleep habits. Include advice on managing stress and relaxation techniques to promote better sleep. Emphasize the significance of seeking professional help if sleep problems persist.

This outline will delve into the essential aspects of sleep and its profound impact on overall health and well-being. Ready to dive into writing any of these points, or something else on your mind?

Sleep is a fundamental physiological process that is essential for our survival and well-being. Despite spending about a third of our lives asleep, many people underestimate the importance of sleep and its complex biological processes. Understanding the science of sleep can help us appreciate its vital role in maintaining health and optimizing daily functioning.

Sleep is not a uniform state but consists of multiple stages that cycle throughout the night. These stages are broadly categorized into Rapid Eye Movement (REM) sleep and Non-Rapid Eye Movement (Non-REM) sleep. Non-REM sleep is further divided into three stages: N1, N2, and N3.

Stage N1: This is the lightest stage of sleep, acting as a transition between wakefulness and sleep. During N1, brain activity begins to slow down, and muscle activity decreases. It is easy to wake up from this stage, and it typically lasts for only a few minutes.

Stage N2: As we move into N2, our body temperature drops, and heart rate slows. This stage constitutes a significant portion of our sleep cycle. Brain activity continues to slow, but there are periodic bursts of rapid brain waves known as sleep spindles. These spindles are thought to play a role in memory consolidation and cognitive processing.

Stage N3: Also known as deep sleep or slow-wave sleep, N3 is characterized by slow brain waves called delta waves. During this stage, the body focuses on physical restoration, including tissue growth and repair, immune system strengthening, and the release of growth hormones. Deep sleep is crucial for feeling refreshed and re-juvenated in the morning.

REM Sleep: REM sleep is distinct from Non-REM sleep and is characterized by rapid eye movements, increased brain activity, and vivid dreaming. During REM sleep, the brain processes emotions, consolidates memories, and enhances cognitive functions. REM sleep is essential for mental and emotional health, and its deficiency can lead to mood disturbances and impaired cognitive performance.

A typical sleep cycle lasts about 90 minutes and consists of a progression through the stages of Non-REM sleep followed by a period of REM sleep. Throughout the night, we typically experience four to six sleep cycles, with the proportion of REM sleep increasing in the latter half of the night.

The regulation of sleep is influenced by our circadian rhythm, an internal biological clock that operates on a roughly 24-hour cycle. The circadian rhythm is governed by the suprachiasmatic nucleus (SCN) in the hypothalamus, which responds to environmental cues such as light and darkness. Exposure to natural light in the morning helps synchronize the circadian rhythm, promoting wakefulness during the day and facilitating sleep at night.

Melatonin, a hormone produced by the pineal gland, plays a crucial role in regulating sleep. As daylight diminishes, the SCN signals the pineal gland to release melatonin, which promotes drowsiness and prepares the body for sleep. Conversely, exposure to artificial light, especially blue light from electronic devices, can interfere with melatonin production and disrupt the circadian rhythm, making it harder to fall asleep.

Understanding the science of sleep highlights the importance of maintaining healthy sleep habits and environments. Adequate sleep supports physical restoration, cognitive functioning, and emotional well-being. It is a dynamic and complex process that is essential for overall health. By prioritizing sleep and aligning our habits with our natural circadian rhythm, we can enhance our quality of life and achieve optimal well-being.

Sleep and Physical Health

Sleep is a critical pillar of physical health, playing an essential role in supporting numerous bodily functions. Adequate sleep allows the body to repair itself, regulate vital processes, and maintain overall well-being. Conversely, sleep deprivation can have detrimental effects on physical health, increasing the risk of chronic conditions and impairing daily functioning.

One of the primary benefits of sleep is its role in supporting the immune system. During sleep, the body produces and releases cytokines, proteins that help combat infection, inflammation, and stress. These cytokines are crucial for immune response, enabling the body to fight off pathogens and recover from illness. Sleep deprivation can reduce the production of these protective proteins, weakening the immune system and making individuals more susceptible to infections, such as the common cold and flu.

Hormone regulation is another critical function of sleep. Various hormones, including growth hormone, cortisol, and insulin, are regulated during sleep. Growth hormone, which is essential for tissue growth and repair, is predominantly secreted during deep sleep. This hormone promotes muscle repair, bone growth, and overall physical recovery. Cortisol, often referred to as the stress hormone, follows a diurnal pattern, with levels peaking in the morning and declining throughout the day. Adequate sleep helps maintain this rhythm, preventing excessive cortisol production, which can lead to stress-related health issues.

Sleep also plays a significant role in metabolic health. Insufficient sleep can disrupt the balance of hunger-regulating hormones, leptin and ghrelin. Leptin signals satiety and reduces appetite, while ghrelin stimulates hunger. Sleep deprivation increases ghrelin levels and decreases leptin levels, leading to increased appetite and cravings, particularly for high-calorie, carbohydrate-rich foods. This hormonal imbalance can contribute to overeating and weight gain, increasing the risk of obesity and related conditions, such as type 2 diabetes.

The cardiovascular system also benefits from adequate sleep. During sleep, heart rate and blood pressure naturally decrease, allowing the heart and blood vessels to rest and recover. Chronic sleep deprivation, however, can lead to increased heart rate and elevated blood pressure, both of which are risk factors for cardiovascular diseases. Studies have shown that individuals who consistently get insufficient sleep are at a higher risk of developing hypertension, coronary artery disease, and stroke. By prioritizing sleep, we can support heart health and reduce the risk of these serious conditions.

Cellular repair and recovery are other vital processes that occur during sleep. Deep sleep stages are particularly important for the repair of muscles, tissues, and cells. The body produces more protein molecules during deep sleep, which are used for repairing damage caused by stress, exercise, and environmental factors such as UV radiation. This cellular repair process is essential for maintaining overall physical health, promoting muscle recovery, and ensuring the proper functioning of various bodily systems.

Sleep deprivation can have immediate and long-term consequences on physical health. In the short term, it can impair coordination, reaction times, and judgment, increasing the risk of accidents and injuries. Over the long term, chronic sleep deprivation is associated with an increased risk of developing chronic conditions such as heart disease, diabetes, obesity, and certain cancers. It can also exacerbate existing health issues, leading to a decline in overall quality of life.

In summary, sleep is a fundamental component of physical health, supporting immune function, hormone regulation, metabolic balance, cardiovascular health, and cellular repair. By prioritizing adequate and quality sleep, we can enhance our physical well-being, reduce the risk of chronic diseases, and improve our overall quality of life. Embrace the power of sleep as an essential part of a healthy lifestyle, and ensure that it remains a top priority in your daily routine.

The connection between sleep and mental health is both profound and bidirectional. Adequate sleep is essential for maintaining mental well-being, and disruptions in sleep can have significant impacts on cognitive function, mood regulation, and emotional resilience. Understanding this relationship can help highlight the importance of prioritizing good sleep hygiene as a fundamental component of mental health care.

Cognitive Functions Sleep plays a crucial role in cognitive processes such as learning, memory, and problem-solving. During sleep, particularly during REM sleep, the brain consolidates and processes the information learned during the day. This process helps strengthen memory and improve recall. Sleep also enhances cognitive functions such as attention, concentration, and decision-making. On the flip side, sleep deprivation can impair these cognitive abilities, leading to difficulties in focusing, decreased productivity, and impaired judgment. Chronic sleep deprivation can exacerbate these issues, making everyday tasks more challenging and increasing the risk of errors and accidents.

Mood Regulation One of the most noticeable effects of sleep on mental health is its impact on mood regulation. Adequate sleep helps stabilize mood and reduces irritability, anxiety, and stress. During sleep, the brain processes emotions and emotional experiences, which helps in managing and regulating feelings. Lack of sleep, however, can lead to increased emotional reactivity, making it harder to cope with stress and negative emotions. This can result in mood swings, heightened anxiety, and a greater susceptibility to stress. Over time, chronic sleep deprivation can contribute to the development of mood disorders such as depression and anxiety.

Emotional Resilience Sleep is essential for emotional resilience—the ability to cope with and recover from life's challenges. Adequate sleep strengthens emotional resilience by enhancing the brain's ability to regulate emotions and respond to stress. It promotes a more positive outlook and helps individuals maintain a sense of balance even in difficult situations. Conversely, insufficient sleep can weaken emotional resilience, making it harder to manage stress, adapt to changes, and recover from setbacks. This can create a cycle where stress and sleep problems reinforce each other, leading to a decline in mental well-being.

Sleep Disorders and Mental Health Conditions There is a bidirectional relationship between sleep disorders and mental health conditions. Conditions such as insomnia, sleep apnea, and restless legs syndrome can significantly impact sleep quality and duration. Insomnia, characterized by difficulty falling or staying asleep, can lead to chronic sleep deprivation and exacerbate mental health issues. Sleep apnea, a condition where breathing repeatedly stops and starts during sleep, can lead to fragmented sleep and daytime fatigue, affecting mood and cognitive function. Restless legs syndrome, which causes an irresistible urge to move the legs, can disrupt sleep and contribute to sleep deprivation.

On the other hand, mental health conditions such as anxiety and depression can disrupt sleep patterns, leading to difficulty falling asleep, staying asleep, or experiencing restful sleep. Anxiety often causes racing thoughts and heightened arousal, making it hard to relax and fall asleep. Depression can lead to changes in sleep patterns, with some individuals experiencing insomnia and others sleeping excessively. Addressing sleep issues is a critical component of managing these mental health conditions and improving overall well-being.

Addressing Sleep Issues to Support Mental Health Improving sleep quality and duration is essential for supporting mental health. Adopting healthy sleep habits, such as maintaining a consistent sleep schedule, creating a relaxing bedtime routine, and optimizing the sleep environment, can promote better sleep. Reducing exposure to blue light from electronic devices before bedtime, avoiding caffeine and heavy meals close to bedtime, and engaging in relaxation techniques such as meditation or deep breathing can also enhance sleep quality.

For individuals with chronic sleep problems or sleep disorders, seeking professional help is important. A healthcare provider can assess and diagnose sleep issues, offering treatments such as cognitive-behavioral therapy for insomnia (CBT-I), continuous positive airway pressure (CPAP) for sleep apnea, or medications if necessary. Addressing underlying mental health conditions through therapy, counseling, or medication can also improve sleep quality and overall mental well-being.

In summary, sleep is a critical component of mental health, influencing cognitive functions, mood regulation, and emotional resilience. Understanding the connection between sleep and mental health highlights the importance of prioritizing good sleep hygiene and seeking professional help for sleep disorders. By fostering healthy sleep habits and addressing sleep issues, we can enhance mental well-being and improve our overall quality of life.

Common Sleep Disorders and Their Management

Sleep disorders are prevalent and can significantly impact an individual's quality of life. These conditions disrupt normal sleep patterns, leading to difficulties in falling asleep, staying asleep, or achieving restorative sleep. Understanding common sleep disorders, their symptoms, and management strategies is crucial for improving sleep health and overall well-being.

Insomnia: Insomnia is one of the most common sleep disorders, characterized by persistent difficulty falling asleep, staying asleep, or waking up too early and being unable to go back to sleep. People with insomnia often experience daytime fatigue, irritability, and difficulties with concentration and memory. Insomnia can be short-term (acute), often triggered by stress or a significant life event, or long-term (chronic), lasting for months or even years. The causes of insomnia vary, including psychological factors such as anxiety and depression, lifestyle factors like irregular sleep schedules and excessive screen time, and medical conditions such as chronic pain or medications.

Management strategies for insomnia focus on improving sleep hygiene and cognitive-behavioral therapy for insomnia (CBT-I). Sleep hygiene involves establishing a regular sleep schedule, creating a restful sleep environment, avoiding caffeine and heavy meals close to bedtime, and limiting exposure to screens before sleep. CBT-I is a structured program that helps individuals identify and change thoughts and behaviors that contribute to insomnia. In some cases, medications may be prescribed, but they are typically considered a short-term solution.

Sleep Apnea Sleep apnea is a serious sleep disorder in which breathing repeatedly stops and starts during sleep. The most common type is obstructive sleep apnea (OSA), where the throat muscles intermittently relax and block the airway. Symptoms of sleep apnea include loud snoring, episodes of stopped breathing witnessed by others, abrupt awakenings accompanied by gasping or choking, and excessive daytime sleepiness. Untreated sleep apnea can lead to severe health issues, including hypertension, heart disease, stroke, and diabetes.

Management of sleep apnea often involves lifestyle changes, such as weight loss, quitting smoking, and sleeping on one's side. Continuous Positive Airway Pressure (CPAP) therapy is a common treatment that involves wearing a mask over the nose and/or mouth during sleep, which delivers a steady stream of air to keep the airway open. Other treatments include oral appliances that reposition the jaw and, in some cases, surgical interventions to remove obstructive tissues or enlarge the airway.

Restless Legs Syndrome (RLS) Restless Legs Syndrome (RLS) is a neurological disorder characterized by an uncontrollable urge to move the legs, usually due to uncomfortable sensations. These sensations often worsen in the evening or at night and can severely disrupt sleep. The exact cause of RLS is not well understood, but it may be linked to an imbalance of dopamine, a brain chemical that controls muscle movement. RLS can also be associated with other conditions such as iron deficiency, kidney failure, or peripheral neuropathy.

Management strategies for RLS include lifestyle changes, such as regular exercise, maintaining a consistent sleep schedule, and avoiding caffeine and alcohol. Medications that affect dopamine levels, as well as supplements for iron deficiency if present, may also be prescribed. Non-pharmacological treatments, such as leg massages, warm baths, and the application of heat or cold packs, can provide relief from symptoms.

Narcolepsy: Narcolepsy is a chronic sleep disorder characterized by overwhelming daytime drowsiness and sudden attacks of sleep. People with narcolepsy may experience cataplexy (sudden loss of muscle tone), sleep paralysis (temporary inability to move or speak while falling asleep or waking up), and hallucinations. Narcolepsy is caused by a deficiency of hypocretin, a brain chemical that regulates wakefulness and REM sleep. The condition can significantly impact daily activities and overall quality of life.

Management of narcolepsy involves a combination of medications and lifestyle changes. Stimulant medications can help maintain wakefulness during the day, while antidepressants may be used to manage cataplexy and other symptoms. Lifestyle modifications, such as maintaining a regular sleep schedule, taking short naps during the day, and avoiding caffeine and alcohol, can help manage symptoms and improve quality of life.

Circadian Rhythm Sleep-Wake Disorders Circadian rhythm sleep-wake disorders occur when there is a misalignment between an individual's internal biological clock and the external environment. Examples include delayed sleep-wake phase disorder (where individuals go to sleep and wake up much later than desired), shift work disorder (caused by irregular work hours), and jet lag (caused by traveling across multiple time zones). These disorders can lead to difficulties in falling asleep, staying asleep, and excessive daytime sleepiness.

Management strategies for circadian rhythm disorders focus on realigning the body's internal clock with the desired sleep-wake schedule. This can be achieved through light therapy, which involves exposure to bright light at specific times to reset the circadian rhythm, and chronotherapy, a gradual adjustment of sleep times. Maintaining a consistent sleep schedule, practicing good sleep hygiene, and, in some cases, using melatonin supplements can also help manage these disorders.

In summary, understanding and managing sleep disorders is essential for improving sleep quality and overall health. By recognizing the symptoms and seeking appropriate treatment, individuals can achieve better sleep and enhance their well-being. Prioritize sleep health and consult healthcare professionals if you suspect a sleep disorder, as effective management can lead to significant improvements in your quality of life.

Strategies for Improving Sleep Quality

Achieving high-quality sleep is essential for overall health and well-being. Good sleep hygiene—habits and practices that promote consistent, uninterrupted sleep—plays a crucial role in enhancing sleep quality. By adopting effective strategies and making intentional changes to your sleep environment and daily routine, you can enjoy more restful and restorative sleep.

Establish a Regular Sleep Routine Consistency is key to good sleep. Going to bed and waking up at the same time every day, including weekends, helps regulate your body's internal clock, known as the circadian rhythm. This regularity makes it easier to fall asleep and wake up naturally. To establish a consistent sleep schedule, determine a bedtime that allows for 7-9 hours of sleep and set an alarm to wake up at the same time each morning. Gradually adjust your sleep schedule by 15-30 minutes each night if needed, rather than making abrupt changes.

Create a Sleep-Conducive Environment Your sleep environment plays a significant role in the quality of your sleep. Aim to create a bedroom that is cool, quiet, and dark. A comfortable mattress and pillows that support your preferred sleep position are essential. Consider using blackout curtains to block out external light and earplugs or a white noise machine to minimize noise disruptions. Keep electronic devices, such as smartphones, tablets, and TVs, out of the bedroom to reduce exposure to blue light, which can interfere with melatonin production and disrupt sleep.

Adopt Healthy Sleep Habits Incorporating healthy habits into your daily routine can promote better sleep. Engage in regular physical activity, such as walking, jogging, or yoga, but avoid vigorous exercise close to bedtime as it may stimulate the body and make it harder to fall asleep. Be mindful of your diet; avoid heavy meals, caffeine, and alcohol in the hours leading up to bedtime. While alcohol may initially make you feel sleepy, it can disrupt your sleep cycle and reduce sleep quality. Opt for a light snack if you're hungry before bed, such as a banana or a handful of nuts.

Manage Stress and Relaxation Stress and anxiety can significantly impact your ability to fall and stay asleep. Developing relaxation techniques can help calm your mind and prepare your body for sleep. Practices such as deep breathing exercises, progressive muscle relaxation, and mindfulness meditation can reduce stress and promote relaxation. Establish a calming bedtime routine to signal to your body that it's time to wind down. This routine might include activities such as reading a book, taking a warm bath, or listening to soothing music. Avoid stimulating activities and bright screens in the hour leading up to bedtime.

Address Sleep Disorders and Seek Professional Help If you have persistent sleep problems or suspect a sleep disorder, it's important to seek professional help. Conditions such as insomnia, sleep apnea, and restless legs syndrome require specific treatments that can significantly improve sleep quality. Cognitive-behavioral therapy for insomnia (CBT-I) is an effective, evidence-based treatment that helps individuals change behaviors and thoughts that interfere with sleep. For sleep apnea, treatments such as Continuous Positive Airway Pressure (CPAP) therapy can alleviate symptoms and improve sleep. Consulting a healthcare provider or a sleep specialist can help diagnose and manage sleep disorders, leading to better sleep and overall health.

In conclusion, improving sleep quality requires a combination of consistent routines, a sleep-conducive environment, healthy lifestyle choices, effective stress management, and professional support when needed. By prioritizing sleep and making these intentional changes, you can achieve more restful and restorative sleep, enhancing your overall well-being. Embrace the power of sleep as a vital component of a healthy lifestyle and enjoy the numerous benefits it brings to your physical and mental health.

Chapter 6: Preventive Healthcare

The Importance of Preventive Healthcare

Summary: Discuss the concept of preventive healthcare and its significance in maintaining health and preventing disease. Highlight the benefits of early detection and intervention, such as reducing the risk of chronic diseases and improving long-term health outcomes. Emphasize the role of regular check-ups, screenings, and vaccinations in preventive care.

Routine Health Screenings and Tests

Summary: Outline essential health screenings and tests that should be a part of regular preventive care. Include information on screenings for blood pressure, cholesterol, diabetes, cancer (such as mammograms and colonoscopies), and bone density. Explain the purpose of each screening, the recommended frequency, and how they help in early detection and management of health conditions.

Vaccinations and Immunizations

Summary: Explore the role of vaccinations and immunizations in preventive healthcare. Discuss the importance of vaccines in protecting against infectious diseases, the concept of herd immunity, and the recommended vaccination schedules for different age groups.

Highlight the benefits of staying up-to-date with vaccines and addressing common misconceptions about vaccination.

Healthy Lifestyle Choices

Summary: Emphasize the impact of lifestyle choices on preventive healthcare. Discuss the importance of a balanced diet, regular physical activity, adequate sleep, and stress management in maintaining health and preventing disease. Provide practical tips for adopting and maintaining healthy habits that contribute to overall well-being.

Preventive Care Across Different Life Stages

Summary: Address how preventive healthcare needs vary across different life stages, from childhood to older adulthood. Provide specific recommendations for preventive measures at each stage, such as well-child visits, adolescent health check-ups, reproductive health care, and screenings for older adults. Highlight the importance of tailored preventive care to address the unique health needs of each age group.

This outline will provide a comprehensive look at preventive healthcare, emphasizing the importance of proactive measures in maintaining health and preventing disease. Ready to dive into writing any of these points, or something else on your mind?

Preventive healthcare is the cornerstone of maintaining health and well-being, focusing on the proactive measures that can be taken to prevent disease and detect health issues early. This approach to healthcare emphasizes the importance of regular check-ups, screenings, and vaccinations to identify potential problems before they become serious. By prioritizing preventive measures, individuals can significantly improve their long-term health outcomes, reduce the risk of chronic diseases, and enhance their quality of life.

One of the primary benefits of preventive healthcare is the early detection of health issues. Regular screenings and check-ups allow healthcare providers to identify conditions such as high blood pressure, high cholesterol, diabetes, and certain cancers at an early stage when they are most treatable. Early intervention can prevent the progression of these conditions, reducing the need for more invasive and costly treatments down the line. For example, detecting high blood pressure early and managing it through lifestyle changes or medication can prevent complications such as heart disease and stroke.

Vaccinations are another critical component of preventive healthcare. Immunizations protect against a range of infectious diseases, from measles and influenza to more severe illnesses like pneumonia and hepatitis. Vaccines not only protect the individual but also contribute to herd immunity, reducing the spread of diseases within the community. Staying up-to-date with recommended vaccinations is essential for protecting both personal and public health.

Regular check-ups and screenings are also an opportunity for healthcare providers to offer personalized advice on maintaining a healthy lifestyle. During these visits, patients can discuss their diet, exercise routine, sleep patterns, and stress levels with their healthcare provider. This holistic approach ensures that all aspects of health are addressed, and patients receive guidance on making positive lifestyle changes. For instance, a healthcare provider might recommend a balanced diet rich in fruits, vegetables, and whole grains to support overall health and prevent conditions like obesity and heart disease.

Preventive healthcare is particularly important for managing chronic diseases. Conditions such as diabetes, heart disease, and asthma require ongoing monitoring and management to prevent complications and maintain quality of life. Regular check-ups allow healthcare providers to track the progress of these conditions, adjust treatment plans as needed, and provide support and education to patients. By closely monitoring their health, individuals with chronic diseases can stay on top of their condition and avoid hospitalizations and other serious complications.

The economic benefits of preventive healthcare should not be overlooked. By preventing diseases and detecting health issues early, individuals can avoid the high costs associated with treating advanced illnesses. Preventive care is often covered by health insurance plans, making it an accessible and cost-effective option for maintaining health. Investing in preventive measures ultimately reduces the financial burden on both individuals and the healthcare system as a whole.

In addition to the physical and economic benefits, preventive healthcare also positively impacts mental and emotional well-being. Knowing that they are taking proactive steps to maintain their health can provide individuals with peace of mind and a sense of control over their well-being. Regular check-ups offer an opportunity to discuss any health concerns or symptoms with a healthcare provider, alleviating anxiety and fostering a trusting patient-provider relationship.

In conclusion, the importance of preventive healthcare cannot be overstated. By emphasizing early detection, vaccinations, and healthy lifestyle choices, preventive care helps individuals maintain optimal health, prevent chronic diseases, and improve their quality of life. Regular check-ups and screenings are essential for catching potential health issues early and providing personalized guidance on maintaining well-being. Embrace preventive healthcare as a fundamental part of your health journey, and reap the benefits of a proactive approach to wellness.

Routine Health Screenings and Tests

Routine health screenings and tests are fundamental components of preventive healthcare, serving as vital tools for early detection and intervention. These screenings can identify health issues before they become serious, allowing for timely treatment and management. By incorporating regular screenings into your healthcare regimen, you can stay proactive about your health and reduce the risk of developing chronic conditions.

Blood Pressure Screening Blood pressure screening is essential for detecting hypertension (high blood pressure), a condition that often presents no symptoms but can lead to serious complications such as heart disease, stroke, and kidney damage. Regular blood pressure checks can help monitor and manage this condition. The American Heart Association recommends that adults have their blood pressure checked at least once every two years if their levels are within the normal range (less than 120/80 mm Hg). If readings are higher, more frequent monitoring may be necessary.

Cholesterol Testing Cholesterol testing, also known as a lipid panel or lipid profile, measures the levels of cholesterol and triglycerides in your blood. High levels of LDL (low-density lipoprotein) cholesterol, often referred to as "bad" cholesterol, can lead to the buildup of plaque in arteries, increasing the risk of heart disease and stroke. HDL (high-density lipoprotein) cholesterol, or "good" cholesterol, helps remove excess cholesterol from the bloodstream. The American Heart Association recommends that adults aged 20 and older have their cholesterol levels checked every four to six years. Those with risk factors for heart disease may need more frequent testing.

Diabetes Screening Diabetes screening is crucial for identifying prediabetes and diabetes, conditions that can cause serious health complications if left untreated. The most common tests for diabetes screening are the fasting blood glucose test, the HbA1c test, and the oral glucose tolerance test (OGTT). The American Diabetes Association recommends that adults aged 45 and older undergo diabetes screening every three years. Individuals with risk factors such as obesity, a family history of diabetes, or a sedentary lifestyle should consider earlier and more frequent testing.

Cancer Screenings Cancer screenings are designed to detect cancer at an early stage when it is most treatable. Common cancer screenings include mammograms for breast cancer, Pap smears and HPV tests for cervical cancer, colonoscopies for colorectal cancer, and prostate-specific antigen (PSA) tests for prostate cancer. Mammograms are recommended every two years for women aged 50 to 74, while women aged 21 to 65 should have a Pap smear every three years. Colonoscopies are generally recommended starting at age 50 and continuing until age 75, with a frequency of every ten years if results are normal. Men should discuss prostate cancer screening with their healthcare provider to determine the appropriate age and frequency based on individual risk factors.

Bone Density Testing Bone density testing, or DEXA (dual-energy X-ray absorptiometry) scan, measures bone mineral density and helps diagnose osteoporosis. Osteoporosis is a condition characterized by weakened bones, increasing the risk of fractures. Bone density testing is particularly important for postmenopausal women and older adults. The National Osteoporosis Foundation recommends that women aged 65 and older and men aged 70 and older undergo bone density testing. Individuals with risk factors such as a family history of osteoporosis, long-term use of corticosteroids, or certain medical conditions may require earlier testing.

Summary Routine health screenings and tests are essential for maintaining health and preventing disease. By regularly monitoring vital health indicators such as blood pressure, cholesterol levels, blood glucose, and bone density, individuals can detect and address potential health issues early. Cancer screenings are critical for early detection and successful treatment of various cancers. Discuss with your healthcare provider which screenings and tests are appropriate for you based on your age, gender, and risk factors. Embrace the proactive approach of preventive healthcare, and prioritize regular screenings to safeguard your health and well-being.

Vaccinations and Immunizations

Vaccinations and immunizations are integral components of preventive healthcare, playing a crucial role in protecting individuals and communities from infectious diseases. By stimulating the immune system to recognize and combat pathogens, vaccines help prevent the spread of contagious illnesses, reduce the incidence of severe disease, and save lives. Understanding the importance of vaccinations, the concept of herd immunity, and the recommended vaccination schedules can help individuals make informed decisions about their health.

Importance of Vaccinations Vaccines are designed to provide immunity against specific diseases by exposing the immune system to a harmless form of the pathogen, such as an inactivated or weakened virus, or a piece of the pathogen, such as a protein. This exposure prompts the immune system to produce antibodies, which are proteins that recognize and neutralize the pathogen. If the vaccinated individual is later exposed to the actual disease-causing pathogen, their immune system is prepared to respond quickly and effectively, preventing illness.

Vaccinations have led to the eradication or significant reduction of many infectious diseases that once caused widespread morbidity and mortality. For example, smallpox, a deadly disease that claimed millions of lives, was eradicated globally through vaccination efforts. Polio, which caused paralysis and death, has been nearly eradicated, with only a few cases reported in a handful of countries. Measles, mumps, rubella, and diphtheria are among other diseases that have seen dramatic declines in incidence due to widespread vaccination.

Herd Immunity Herd immunity occurs when a significant portion of a population becomes immune to a contagious disease, either through vaccination or previous infection, reducing the likelihood of disease spread. This protection is especially important for individuals who cannot be vaccinated due to medical reasons, such as those with compromised immune systems or severe allergies to vaccine components. When a large percentage of the population is immune, the spread of the disease is limited, providing indirect protection to vulnerable individuals.

Achieving herd immunity through vaccination is a cornerstone of public health efforts to control and eliminate infectious diseases. It requires high vaccination coverage to ensure that enough people are immune to interrupt the transmission of the pathogen. Herd immunity thresholds vary depending on the disease and its mode of transmission, but generally, coverage rates of 70-95% are needed to achieve herd immunity for most vaccine-preventable diseases.

Recommended Vaccination Schedules Vaccination schedules are developed by public health organizations and medical experts based on evidence of vaccine safety and efficacy. These schedules outline the recommended ages and intervals for administering vaccines to provide optimal protection throughout life. Key vaccines and their recommended schedules include:

Childhood Vaccines: Children should receive vaccines for diseases such as hepatitis B, rotavirus, diphtheria, tetanus, pertussis (whooping cough), Haemophilus influenzae type b (Hib), pneumococcal disease, polio, influenza, measles, mumps, rubella, varicella (chickenpox), and hepatitis A. The immunization schedule typically begins at birth and continues through adolescence, with booster doses administered as needed.

Adolescent Vaccines: Adolescents should receive vaccines such as the human papillomavirus (HPV) vaccine, which protects against cancers caused by HPV infection, and the meningococcal vaccine, which protects against meningococcal disease. Booster doses of tetanus, diphtheria, and pertussis (Tdap) are also recommended during adolescence.

Adult Vaccines: Adults should stay up-to-date with vaccines such as the influenza vaccine, administered annually to protect against seasonal flu, and the Tdap booster every 10 years. Other vaccines, such as the shingles vaccine (recommended for adults aged 50 and older) and the pneumococcal vaccine (recommended for adults aged 65 and older), are important for preventing specific diseases in older adults.

Special Populations: Individuals with certain medical conditions, travelers, and healthcare workers may require additional vaccines or earlier vaccination schedules. For example, healthcare workers should receive the hepatitis B vaccine and annual influenza vaccine to protect themselves and their patients. Travelers may need vaccines such as the yellow fever or typhoid vaccine, depending on their destination.

Addressing Common Misconceptions Despite the overwhelming evidence supporting the safety and efficacy of vaccines, misconceptions and misinformation can create hesitation or resistance to vaccination. Common myths include the false belief that vaccines cause autism, that natural immunity is better than vaccine-induced immunity, or that vaccine-preventable diseases are no longer a threat. It is important to address these misconceptions with accurate information from reputable sources. Vaccines undergo rigorous testing and monitoring to ensure their safety and effectiveness, and the benefits of vaccination far outweigh the risks.

In conclusion, vaccinations and immunizations are essential for preventing infectious diseases, achieving herd immunity, and protecting public health. By following recommended vaccination schedules and addressing common misconceptions, individuals can make informed decisions to safeguard their health and the health of their communities. Embrace the power of vaccines as a critical component of preventive healthcare, and contribute to a healthier and safer world for everyone.

Healthy Lifestyle Choices

Adopting healthy lifestyle choices is a cornerstone of preventive healthcare. By making intentional decisions about diet, physical activity, sleep, and stress management, individuals can significantly improve their overall health and reduce the risk of developing chronic diseases. Here's how to integrate these choices into your daily routine to support long-term well-being.

Balanced Diet A balanced diet is essential for providing the nutrients your body needs to function optimally. It involves consuming a variety of foods from all food groups in the right proportions. Aim to fill half your plate with fruits and vegetables, which are rich in vitamins, minerals, and antioxidants that support overall health. Choose whole grains like brown rice, quinoa, and whole wheat bread over refined grains to ensure you get enough fiber and nutrients.

Incorporate lean proteins such as chicken, fish, beans, and legumes to support muscle health and repair. Healthy fats, found in sources like avocados, nuts, seeds, and olive oil, are crucial for brain health and hormone production. Limit the intake of saturated fats, trans fats, added sugars, and sodium, which can contribute to heart disease, obesity, and other health issues. Staying hydrated by drinking plenty of water is also vital for maintaining bodily functions.

Regular Physical Activity Engaging in regular physical activity is one of the most effective ways to prevent chronic diseases and promote overall health. Aim for at least 150 minutes of moderate-intensity aerobic exercise, such as brisk walking, cycling, or swimming, each week. Alternatively, 75 minutes of vigorous-intensity aerobic exercise, like running or high-intensity interval training (HIIT), can provide similar benefits.

In addition to aerobic exercise, include strength training activities at least two days a week to build and maintain muscle mass and bone density. Exercises like weightlifting, resistance band workouts, and bodyweight exercises such as push-ups and squats are effective options. Flexibility and balance exercises, such as yoga and Tai Chi, are also important for maintaining mobility and reducing the risk of falls, especially as you age.

Adequate Sleep Quality sleep is essential for physical and mental health. Adults should aim for 7-9 hours of sleep per night. Establishing a regular sleep schedule by going to bed and waking up at the same time each day helps regulate your body's internal clock. Create a relaxing bedtime routine to signal to your body that it's time to wind down. This might include activities like reading, taking a warm bath, or practicing deep breathing exercises.

Optimize your sleep environment by keeping your bedroom cool, dark, and quiet. Invest in a comfortable mattress and pillows, and remove electronic devices that emit blue light, which can interfere with melatonin production. If you have trouble sleeping, consider lifestyle changes such as reducing caffeine intake, especially in the afternoon and evening, and avoiding large meals close to bedtime.

Stress Management Chronic stress can have detrimental effects on physical and mental health, contributing to conditions such as heart disease, depression, and anxiety. Developing effective stress management techniques is crucial for maintaining well-being. Mindfulness practices, such as meditation, deep breathing exercises, and progressive muscle relaxation, can help reduce stress and promote a sense of calm.

Time management strategies, such as prioritizing tasks, setting realistic goals, and taking regular breaks, can also alleviate stress. Engage in activities that bring you joy and relaxation, whether it's spending time in nature, pursuing a hobby, or connecting with loved ones. Social support is vital for managing stress, so make time to nurture relationships and seek help when needed.

Avoiding Harmful Behaviors In addition to adopting positive lifestyle habits, it's important to avoid behaviors that can negatively impact health. This includes smoking cessation, limiting alcohol consumption, and avoiding the misuse of drugs. Smoking is a leading cause of preventable diseases, including cancer, heart disease, and respiratory conditions. Quitting smoking can significantly improve health outcomes and reduce the risk of chronic diseases.

Moderate alcohol consumption, defined as up to one drink per day for women and up to two drinks per day for men, can be part of a healthy lifestyle. However, excessive drinking can lead to liver disease, cardiovascular problems, and other health issues. If you choose to drink, do so responsibly and be aware of the potential risks.

In conclusion, making healthy lifestyle choices is a powerful way to support preventive healthcare and enhance overall well-being. By focusing on a balanced diet, regular physical activity, adequate sleep, stress management, and avoiding harmful behaviors, you can take proactive steps to prevent chronic diseases and maintain good health. Embrace these habits as part of your daily routine and enjoy the benefits of a healthier, more fulfilling life.

Preventive Care Across Different Life Stages

Preventive healthcare needs vary significantly across different stages of life, and understanding these variations is essential for maintaining health and well-being throughout the lifespan. By tailoring preventive measures to the unique health requirements of each age group, individuals can proactively manage their health and reduce the risk of disease.

Childhood In childhood, preventive care focuses on promoting growth, development, and early detection of potential health issues. Well-child visits are a cornerstone of pediatric preventive care, allowing healthcare providers to monitor physical and developmental milestones, administer vaccinations, and provide guidance on nutrition and safety. During these visits, children receive essential immunizations to protect against infectious diseases such as measles, mumps, rubella, and pertussis. Regular screenings for vision, hearing, and dental health are also important during this stage. Parents and caregivers play a crucial role in establishing healthy habits, such as balanced nutrition, physical activity, and adequate sleep, which lay the foundation for lifelong health.

Adolescence During adolescence, preventive care focuses on addressing the physical, emotional, and social changes that occur during this period of rapid growth and development. Routine health check-ups provide an opportunity to screen for conditions such as obesity, anemia, and mental health issues. Vaccinations remain essential, with additional vaccines such as the human papillomavirus (HPV) vaccine, which protects against certain cancers, and the meningococcal vaccine, which prevents meningococcal disease.

Adolescents should also receive education on topics such as sexual health, substance abuse, and mental well-being. Encouraging healthy behaviors, such as regular exercise, balanced nutrition, and stress management, is crucial for establishing habits that support long-term health.

Adulthood In adulthood, preventive care focuses on maintaining health, detecting early signs of chronic diseases, and addressing lifestyle factors that impact well-being. Regular health check-ups, including screenings for blood pressure, cholesterol, diabetes, and certain cancers, are essential for early detection and management of health conditions. Women should undergo regular Pap smears and mammograms, while men should consider prostate cancer screenings based on individual risk factors. Vaccinations, such as the influenza vaccine and Tdap booster, remain important for protecting against infectious diseases. Adopting a healthy lifestyle, including a balanced diet, regular physical activity, adequate sleep, and stress management, is key to preventing chronic diseases such as heart disease, diabetes, and cancer.

Older Adulthood As individuals age, preventive care becomes increasingly important for managing the risk of chronic diseases and maintaining quality of life. Older adults should have regular screenings for conditions such as osteoporosis, vision and hearing loss, and cognitive decline. Vaccinations, such as the shingles vaccine and pneumococcal vaccine, are critical for protecting against illnesses that can have severe consequences in older age. Managing multiple chronic conditions often becomes a focus of preventive care, with an emphasis on medication management, regular monitoring, and lifestyle modifications. Preventing falls and maintaining mobility through exercises that improve balance and strength are also important for reducing the risk of injury and promoting independence.

Reproductive Health Reproductive health is a critical aspect of preventive care that spans different life stages. For women, preventive care includes regular gynecological exams, screenings for sexually transmitted infections (STIs), and prenatal care during pregnancy. Contraceptive counseling and family planning services help individuals make informed decisions about their reproductive health. Men should also receive screenings for STIs and discuss reproductive health concerns with their healthcare provider. Ensuring access to reproductive health services and education supports overall well-being and empowers individuals to make choices that align with their health goals.

In summary, preventive care is a dynamic and lifelong process that evolves with the changing health needs of each life stage. By prioritizing regular health check-ups, screenings, vaccinations, and healthy lifestyle choices, individuals can proactively manage their health and reduce the risk of disease. Tailoring preventive measures to the unique requirements of each age group ensures comprehensive care and promotes long-term well-being. Embrace preventive healthcare as a fundamental part of your health journey, and stay proactive in maintaining your health at every stage of life.

Chapter 7: Managing Chronic Conditions

Understanding Chronic Conditions

Summary: Define what chronic conditions are and discuss their prevalence and impact on individuals and healthcare systems. Highlight common chronic conditions such as diabetes, hypertension, heart disease, and arthritis. Discuss the importance of early diagnosis and ongoing management to improve quality of life and prevent complications.

Developing a Comprehensive Management Plan

Summary: Outline the components of an effective management plan for chronic conditions. Discuss the role of healthcare providers, medication management, lifestyle modifications, and regular monitoring. Emphasize the importance of individualized care plans tailored to each patient's specific needs and conditions.

Lifestyle Modifications and Self-Care Practices

Summary: Explore the lifestyle changes and self-care practices that can help manage chronic conditions. Include information on diet, exercise, stress management, and smoking cessation. Provide practical tips for incorporating these changes into daily life and highlight the benefits of patient education and support groups.

Medication Management and Adherence

Summary: Discuss the role of medications in managing chronic conditions. Explain the importance of medication adherence and strategies for ensuring patients take their medications as prescribed. Address common barriers to adherence, such as side effects and cost, and provide solutions to overcome these challenges.

The Role of Technology in Chronic Condition Management

Summary: Examine how technology can support the management of chronic conditions. Discuss the use of telemedicine, mobile health apps, wearable devices, and remote monitoring. Highlight the benefits of technology in improving patient engagement, adherence, and overall health outcomes.

This outline covers a comprehensive approach to managing chronic conditions, emphasizing early diagnosis, personalized care, lifestyle modifications, medication adherence, and the role of technology. Ready to dive into writing any of these points, or something else in mind?

Chronic conditions are long-lasting health issues that persist for a year or more and require ongoing medical attention or limit daily activities, or both. These conditions, such as diabetes, hypertension, heart disease, and arthritis, have a profound impact on individuals' lives and the healthcare system as a whole. Understanding what chronic conditions are, their prevalence, and their implications is crucial for improving health outcomes and enhancing the quality of life for those affected.

Chronic conditions are often characterized by their persistence and the need for continuous management. Unlike acute conditions, which typically resolve within a short period, chronic conditions can last for an extended period, sometimes for a lifetime. They often develop slowly and may not exhibit symptoms initially, making early detection and diagnosis challenging. However, once diagnosed, these conditions require regular monitoring, lifestyle adjustments, and sometimes long-term medication to manage effectively.

The prevalence of chronic conditions is on the rise globally, driven by factors such as aging populations, unhealthy lifestyles, and environmental changes. According to the World Health Organization (WHO), chronic diseases are responsible for 71% of all deaths worldwide. In the United States, the Centers for Disease Control and Prevention (CDC) reports that six in ten adults have at least one chronic disease, and four in ten adults have two or more. The most common chronic conditions include heart disease, cancer, chronic lung disease, stroke, Alzheimer's disease, diabetes, and chronic kidney disease.

Diabetes is a prime example of a chronic condition that requires meticulous management. It occurs when the body either cannot produce enough insulin (Type 1 diabetes) or cannot use insulin effectively (Type 2 diabetes). This leads to elevated blood sugar levels, which can cause severe complications such as heart disease, kidney damage, nerve damage, and vision loss. Managing diabetes involves regular blood sugar monitoring, medication, dietary changes, and physical activity to maintain blood sugar levels within a target range.

Hypertension, or high blood pressure, is another prevalent chronic condition. It occurs when the force of blood against the artery walls is consistently too high, which can lead to heart disease, stroke, and kidney failure. Often termed the "silent killer" due to its lack of symptoms, hypertension requires regular monitoring and management through lifestyle changes such as a low-sodium diet, regular exercise, and medication adherence to reduce the risk of complications.

Heart disease encompasses a range of conditions affecting the heart, including coronary artery disease, heart failure, and arrhythmias. It is the leading cause of death worldwide, making its management critical. Preventive measures, early detection, and continuous management through lifestyle changes and medications are essential for reducing the burden of heart disease and improving patient outcomes.

Arthritis, a condition characterized by inflammation of the joints, can significantly impact an individual's quality of life by causing pain, stiffness, and decreased mobility. Osteoarthritis and rheumatoid arthritis are the two most common types. Management strategies include physical therapy, medications to reduce inflammation and pain, and lifestyle changes such as maintaining a healthy weight and engaging in low-impact exercises to preserve joint function.

The importance of early diagnosis and ongoing management of chronic conditions cannot be overstated. Early detection allows for timely intervention, which can slow disease progression, reduce the risk of complications, and improve overall quality of life. Regular check-ups, screenings, and awareness of risk factors are critical components of preventive care. Once diagnosed, a comprehensive management plan tailored to the individual's specific needs and conditions is essential for effective disease management.

In summary, understanding chronic conditions and their impact is vital for improving health outcomes and enhancing the quality of life for those affected. By recognizing the prevalence and implications of chronic conditions such as diabetes, hypertension, heart disease, and arthritis, and emphasizing the importance of early diagnosis and ongoing management, individuals can take proactive steps to manage their health and prevent complications. Embrace a proactive approach to chronic condition management, and work closely with healthcare providers to develop and maintain effective care plans.

Developing a Comprehensive Management Plan

Effectively managing chronic conditions requires a comprehensive and individualized approach that addresses all aspects of the disease and its impact on the patient's life. A well-structured management plan involves collaboration between healthcare providers, patients, and sometimes caregivers, ensuring that all elements of care are coordinated and optimized. Here's how to develop and implement a comprehensive management plan for chronic conditions.

Role of Healthcare Providers Healthcare providers, including primary care physicians, specialists, nurses, and allied health professionals, play a critical role in the management of chronic conditions. They are responsible for diagnosing the condition, developing a treatment plan, monitoring progress, and making necessary adjustments. Regular follow-up appointments are essential for assessing the effectiveness of the treatment plan, identifying any new symptoms or complications, and addressing concerns. Open communication between the patient and healthcare providers is crucial for building trust and ensuring that the patient feels supported and informed throughout their care journey.

Medication Management Medications are often a central component of managing chronic conditions. They can help control symptoms, slow disease progression, and prevent complications. For example, patients with hypertension may be prescribed antihypertensive medications to lower blood pressure, while those with diabetes may require insulin or oral hypoglycemic agents to manage blood sugar levels. It's important for patients to understand their medications, including the dosage, timing, and potential side effects. Healthcare providers should provide clear instructions and educate patients on the importance of medication adherence. Using tools such as pill organizers, medication reminders, and smartphone apps can help patients take their medications consistently and correctly.

Lifestyle Modifications Lifestyle modifications are a cornerstone of managing chronic conditions and can have a significant impact on health outcomes. Key areas to focus on include diet, physical activity, stress management, and smoking cessation. A balanced diet rich in fruits, vegetables, whole grains, lean proteins, and healthy fats can help manage conditions such as diabetes, heart disease, and hypertension. Patients should work with healthcare providers or dietitians to develop personalized meal plans that meet their nutritional needs and support their health goals.

Regular physical activity is vital for maintaining overall health and managing chronic conditions. Exercise can help control weight, improve cardiovascular health, enhance mood, and increase energy levels. Patients should aim for at least 150 minutes of moderate-intensity aerobic exercise per week, along with strength training exercises on two or more days per week. It's important to choose activities that the patient enjoys and can maintain long-term.

Stress management is another critical component of chronic condition management. Chronic stress can exacerbate symptoms and negatively impact overall health. Techniques such as mindfulness meditation, deep breathing exercises, yoga, and engaging in hobbies can help reduce stress levels and improve mental well-being. Healthcare providers can offer resources and support for stress management, including referrals to mental health professionals if needed.

Regular Monitoring Regular monitoring is essential for tracking the progress of chronic conditions and making necessary adjustments to the management plan. This can involve routine lab tests, such as blood glucose monitoring for diabetes or lipid panels for heart disease, as well as regular physical exams and imaging studies. Patients should be encouraged to keep track of their health metrics, such as blood pressure, weight, and symptom diaries, and share this information with their healthcare providers during appointments.

Remote monitoring tools, such as wearable devices and mobile health apps, can facilitate real-time tracking and data sharing, allowing for more proactive and personalized care.

Individualized Care Plans Every patient is unique, and a one-size-fits-all approach does not work for managing chronic conditions. Individualized care plans should be tailored to the specific needs, preferences, and circumstances of each patient. This includes considering factors such as age, comorbidities, lifestyle, and social support systems. Healthcare providers should work closely with patients to set realistic and achievable goals, identify potential barriers to adherence, and develop strategies to overcome these challenges. Patient education and empowerment are key components of individualized care, helping patients take an active role in managing their condition and making informed decisions about their health.

In conclusion, developing a comprehensive management plan for chronic conditions involves a multifaceted approach that includes the collaboration of healthcare providers, medication management, lifestyle modifications, regular monitoring, and individualized care plans. By addressing all aspects of the disease and its impact on the patient's life, a well-structured management plan can improve health outcomes, enhance quality of life, and reduce the risk of complications. Embrace this holistic approach to chronic condition management, and work closely with your healthcare team to achieve optimal health and well-being.

Lifestyle Modifications and Self-Care Practices

Managing chronic conditions effectively often hinges on making key lifestyle modifications and embracing self-care practices. These changes can significantly improve health outcomes, enhance quality of life, and empower individuals to take control of their condition.

Here's a deeper dive into how diet, exercise, stress management, and other self-care practices can support the management of chronic conditions.

Diet and Nutrition Diet plays a crucial role in managing chronic conditions such as diabetes, heart disease, and hypertension. Adopting a balanced and nutritious diet can help control symptoms, prevent complications, and improve overall health. Focus on incorporating a variety of fruits, vegetables, whole grains, lean proteins, and healthy fats into your meals. These foods provide essential nutrients, fiber, and antioxidants that support bodily functions and reduce inflammation.

For individuals with diabetes, monitoring carbohydrate intake is vital to managing blood sugar levels. Choose complex carbohydrates, such as whole grains, legumes, and vegetables, over refined sugars and processed foods. These options have a lower glycemic index and provide a slower, more stable release of glucose into the bloodstream.

Heart-healthy diets, such as the Mediterranean diet, emphasize the consumption of healthy fats, including those found in olive oil, nuts, and fatty fish. These fats can help reduce LDL cholesterol levels and decrease the risk of heart disease. Limiting sodium intake is also crucial for managing hypertension. Choose fresh, unprocessed foods whenever possible, and use herbs and spices to enhance flavor without adding salt.

Physical Activity Regular physical activity is essential for managing chronic conditions and improving overall well-being. Exercise helps control weight, improve cardiovascular health, enhance insulin sensitivity, and boost mood. Aim for at least 150 minutes of moderate-intensity aerobic exercise each week, such as brisk walking, cycling, or swimming. Alternatively, 75 minutes of vigorous-intensity exercise, like running or high-intensity interval training (HIIT), can provide similar benefits.

Incorporate strength training exercises at least twice a week to build and maintain muscle mass and bone density. Activities such as weightlifting, resistance band exercises, and bodyweight exercises like push-ups and squats are effective options. Flexibility and balance exercises, such as yoga and Tai Chi, can help improve mobility and reduce the risk of falls, especially for older adults.

It's important to choose physical activities that you enjoy and can sustain long-term. Consult with your healthcare provider before starting a new exercise program, especially if you have any medical concerns or limitations.

Stress Management Chronic stress can exacerbate symptoms and negatively impact overall health, making stress management a critical component of chronic condition management. Developing effective stress reduction techniques can help you maintain emotional balance and improve your quality of life.

Mindfulness practices, such as meditation, deep breathing exercises, and progressive muscle relaxation, can help reduce stress and promote a sense of calm. Engage in activities that bring you joy and relaxation, whether it's spending time in nature, pursuing a hobby, or connecting with loved ones. Social support is vital for managing stress, so make time to nurture relationships and seek help when needed.

Smoking Cessation If you smoke, quitting is one of the most important steps you can take to improve your health and manage chronic conditions. Smoking contributes to a wide range of health issues, including heart disease, respiratory conditions, and cancer. It can also interfere with the effectiveness of certain medications and exacerbate symptoms of chronic conditions.

Seek support from healthcare providers, smoking cessation programs, and support groups to help you quit. Nicotine replacement therapy, medications, and behavioral counseling can increase your chances of success. Remember, it's never too late to quit, and the benefits of quitting smoking begin almost immediately.

Patient Education and Support Groups Education and support are key components of successful chronic condition management. Understanding your condition, treatment options, and self-care practices empowers you to take an active role in your health. Healthcare providers can offer valuable information and resources to help you manage your condition effectively.

Joining support groups, either in-person or online, can provide emotional support, practical advice, and a sense of community. Connecting with others who are facing similar challenges can help reduce feelings of isolation and provide motivation and encouragement. Support groups offer a platform to share experiences, learn from others, and build lasting friendships.

In conclusion, lifestyle modifications and self-care practices are essential for managing chronic conditions and improving overall health. By adopting a balanced diet, engaging in regular physical activity, managing stress, quitting smoking, and seeking education and support, you can take control of your condition and enhance your quality of life. Embrace these changes as part of your daily routine, and work closely with your healthcare team to achieve optimal health and well-being.

Medication Management and Adherence

Medications play a vital role in managing chronic conditions, helping to control symptoms, prevent complications, and improve quality of life. However, the effectiveness of medications largely depends on proper management and adherence. Understanding the importance of medication adherence, addressing common barriers, and implementing strategies to ensure patients take their medications as prescribed are crucial for optimal health outcomes.

The Role of Medications: Medications are often an integral part of the treatment plan for chronic conditions such as diabetes, hypertension, heart disease, and asthma. They can help regulate blood sugar levels, lower blood pressure, reduce cholesterol, and control symptoms such as pain or inflammation. For instance, insulin and oral hypoglycemic agents are essential for managing diabetes, while antihypertensives are critical for controlling high blood pressure. By taking medications as prescribed, patients can achieve better control of their condition and reduce the risk of complications such as heart attacks, strokes, kidney failure, and vision loss.

Importance of Adherence Medication adherence refers to taking medications exactly as prescribed by the healthcare provider, including the correct dosage, timing, and frequency. Adherence is essential for the medications to work effectively and for the patient to achieve the desired health outcomes. Non-adherence can lead to poor disease control, progression of the condition, increased healthcare costs, and a higher risk of hospitalization and mortality. For example, skipping doses of antihypertensive medications can result in uncontrolled blood pressure, increasing the risk of heart attack and stroke.

Common Barriers to Adherence Several factors can contribute to medication non-adherence, including forgetfulness, complexity of the medication regimen, side effects, cost, and lack of understanding of the medication's importance. Patients may forget to take their medications, especially if they have multiple prescriptions with different dosing schedules. Complex regimens can be confusing and difficult to follow. Side effects can be discouraging, leading some patients to stop taking their medications. Financial constraints may also prevent patients from filling their prescriptions. Additionally, a lack of understanding about the medication's role in managing the condition can result in patients not prioritizing their adherence.

Strategies for Improving Adherence Addressing these barriers requires a multifaceted approach and collaboration between healthcare providers, patients, and caregivers. Here are some strategies to improve medication adherence:

Education and Communication: Educating patients about their condition and the importance of their medications is fundamental. Healthcare providers should clearly explain how the medications work, the expected benefits, and the potential side effects. Open communication allows patients to ask questions and express any concerns they may have. Patients should be encouraged to discuss any difficulties they encounter with their medications, so that healthcare providers can offer solutions.

Simplifying Medication Regimens: Simplifying the medication regimen can make it easier for patients to adhere to their treatment plan. This may involve prescribing medications with fewer doses per day or using combination medications that reduce the number of pills taken. Providers should consider the patient's lifestyle and preferences when designing the regimen.

Using Reminders and Tools: Various tools and technologies can help patients remember to take their medications. These include pill organizers, medication reminder apps, and alarm clocks. Some patients may benefit from automated medication dispensers that provide the correct dose at the scheduled time. These tools can help reduce forgetfulness and ensure consistency in medication-taking.

Managing Side Effects: Addressing side effects promptly can improve adherence. Healthcare providers should discuss potential side effects with patients and provide strategies to manage them. If side effects become bothersome, providers can adjust the dosage or switch to a different medication. Patients should be encouraged to report any adverse effects so that appropriate adjustments can be made.

Financial Assistance: Cost can be a significant barrier to medication adherence. Healthcare providers can help by prescribing generic medications, which are often more affordable. Additionally, patients can be directed to patient assistance programs, co-pay cards, and other resources that offer financial support. Pharmacists can also play a role in identifying cost-effective alternatives and providing information on discount programs.

Monitoring and Follow-Up: Regular follow-up appointments allow healthcare providers to monitor the patient's progress, assess adherence, and make necessary adjustments to the treatment plan. During these visits, providers can reinforce the importance of adherence and address any new challenges that arise. Telehealth and remote monitoring tools can facilitate more frequent check-ins and provide additional support.

In conclusion, medication management and adherence are critical components of managing chronic conditions and achieving optimal health outcomes. By understanding the importance of adherence, addressing common barriers, and implementing effective strategies, patients can improve their medication-taking behaviors and better manage their condition. Collaboration between healthcare providers, patients, and caregivers is essential for ensuring adherence and enhancing overall well-being. Embrace these practices as part of your chronic condition management plan, and work closely with your healthcare team to achieve the best possible health outcomes.

The Role of Technology in Chronic Condition Management

Technology has revolutionized the management of chronic conditions, offering innovative solutions that enhance patient care, improve health outcomes, and increase patient engagement. From telemedicine and mobile health apps to wearable devices and remote monitoring systems, technology provides valuable tools for managing chronic conditions effectively and efficiently.

Telemedicine: Telemedicine has emerged as a powerful tool for managing chronic conditions, especially in the wake of the COVID-19 pandemic. It allows patients to connect with healthcare providers remotely through video calls, phone consultations, and secure messaging platforms. Telemedicine offers numerous benefits, including increased access to care, convenience, and reduced need for in-person visits, which can be particularly beneficial for patients with mobility issues or those living in remote areas.

For chronic condition management, telemedicine enables regular follow-up appointments, medication adjustments, and monitoring of symptoms without the need for travel. Patients can discuss their concerns, receive personalized advice, and maintain continuous communication with their healthcare team. Telemedicine also facilitates timely interventions, as healthcare providers can quickly address any changes in the patient's condition and adjust treatment plans as needed.

Mobile Health Apps Mobile health apps, also known as mHealth apps, are designed to help patients manage their chronic conditions by providing access to health information, tracking tools, and personalized recommendations. These apps can monitor various health metrics such as blood sugar levels, blood pressure, medication adherence, and physical activity. They often include features such as reminders, educational resources, and data visualization, empowering patients to take an active role in their health management.

For example, diabetes management apps can help patients log their blood glucose readings, track their carbohydrate intake, and receive feedback on their progress. Similarly, hypertension management apps can monitor blood pressure readings, provide medication reminders, and offer tips for maintaining a healthy lifestyle. These apps enhance patient engagement and enable self-management, leading to better adherence and improved health outcomes.

Wearable Devices Wearable devices, such as fitness trackers, smartwatches, and continuous glucose monitors (CGMs), provide real-time data on various health parameters. These devices can track physical activity, heart rate, sleep patterns, and other vital signs, offering valuable insights into the patient's health status. For chronic condition management, wearable devices enable continuous monitoring, early detection of potential issues, and personalized feedback.

Continuous glucose monitors, for instance, are particularly beneficial for patients with diabetes, as they provide real-time glucose readings and alerts for hypo- or hyperglycemia. Fitness trackers can motivate patients to stay active by setting goals and tracking their progress. Wearable devices enhance patient awareness and engagement, allowing for more proactive and informed decision-making.

Remote Monitoring Systems Remote monitoring systems leverage technology to collect and transmit health data from patients to healthcare providers in real-time. These systems can monitor various chronic conditions, including heart disease, COPD, and diabetes, allowing for continuous assessment and timely interventions. Remote monitoring devices, such as blood pressure monitors, pulse oximeters, and weight scales, transmit data to healthcare providers, who can analyze the information and make necessary adjustments to the treatment plan.

Remote monitoring reduces the need for frequent in-person visits, as healthcare providers can monitor the patient's condition remotely and identify any concerning trends or changes. This approach enhances patient safety, improves disease management, and reduces the risk of complications. It also provides peace of mind for patients, knowing that their health is being closely monitored by their healthcare team.

Patient Engagement and Education Technology plays a crucial role in enhancing patient engagement and education, which are essential for effective chronic condition management. Online platforms, educational websites, and social media provide access to a wealth of information on various chronic conditions, treatment options, and self-care practices. Patients can participate in virtual support groups, access educational videos, and read articles that help them better understand their condition and treatment plan.

Interactive tools, such as quizzes and decision aids, can help patients assess their knowledge, make informed choices, and actively participate in their care. Gamification elements, such as challenges and rewards, can motivate patients to adhere to their treatment plan and maintain healthy behaviors. By leveraging technology, patients become more empowered and engaged in their health management, leading to better adherence and outcomes.

In conclusion, technology has transformed the management of chronic conditions by providing innovative tools and solutions that enhance patient care and engagement. Telemedicine, mobile health apps, wearable devices, and remote monitoring systems offer valuable support for managing chronic conditions effectively. By embracing these technologies, patients can take an active role in their health, improve adherence, and achieve better health outcomes. Work closely with your healthcare team to explore and utilize these technological advancements, and experience the benefits of modern chronic condition management.

Chapter 8: Building Healthy Habits

The Psychology of Habit Formation

Summary: Delve into the science of how habits are formed. Discuss the habit loop, which includes the cue, routine, and reward. Explain how understanding this process can help in developing new healthy habits and breaking old, unhealthy ones. Highlight the role of consistency and repetition in solidifying new behaviors.

Setting Realistic and Achievable Goals

Summary: Discuss the importance of setting SMART goals (Specific, Measurable, Achievable, Relevant, Time-bound) for building healthy habits. Explain how to break down larger goals into smaller, manageable steps. Provide examples of realistic goals and how to track progress to stay motivated and on track.

Creating a Supportive Environment

Summary: Explore how the environment influences habit formation and maintenance. Discuss strategies for creating a physical and social environment that supports healthy habits, such as organizing your space, surrounding yourself with supportive people, and reducing exposure to triggers of unhealthy behaviors. Highlight the importance of community and accountability.

Overcoming Barriers and Staying Motivated

Summary: Identify common barriers to building and maintaining healthy habits, such as lack of time, motivation, and resources. Provide strategies for overcoming these obstacles, including time management, finding intrinsic motivation, and seeking support. Discuss techniques for staying motivated, such as celebrating small wins and maintaining a positive mindset.

Long-Term Maintenance and Adaptation

Summary: Discuss the importance of maintaining healthy habits over the long term and being adaptable to change. Explain how to integrate habits into your lifestyle permanently, and the importance of flexibility in adjusting habits as life circumstances change. Highlight the role of regular self-reflection and reassessment in sustaining healthy behaviors.

This outline covers the key aspects of building healthy habits, emphasizing the psychology behind habit formation, goal setting, creating a supportive environment, overcoming barriers, and maintaining habits over the long term. Ready to dive into writing any of these points, or something else in mind?

Building healthy habits is essential for maintaining well-being and achieving long-term health goals. To develop and sustain these habits, it's crucial to understand the psychology of habit formation, including the mechanisms that drive our behaviors and the strategies that can help us create positive changes.

At the heart of habit formation lies the habit loop, a three-step process that includes the cue, routine, and reward. Understanding this loop can provide valuable insights into how habits are formed and how we can leverage this knowledge to establish new, healthy behaviors.

Cue: The Trigger The cue is a trigger that initiates the habit loop. It can be an external event, such as seeing a friend go for a run, or an internal state, like feeling stressed or hungry. Cues play a pivotal role in signaling our brains to start a particular behavior. For example, the sight of a toothbrush in the bathroom acts as a cue to brush our teeth. Identifying and recognizing the cues that trigger your habits is the first step in understanding and modifying them.

Routine: The Behavior The routine is the behavior or action that follows the cue. It's the habit itself, whether it's a morning jog, a late-night snack, or checking social media. Routines can be physical actions, mental activities, or emotional responses. Consistency in performing the routine is key to habit formation. Repetition reinforces the behavior, making it more automatic over time. To build a new healthy habit, it's important to choose a routine that is achievable and sustainable. Start small and gradually build up to more significant changes.

Reward: The Benefit The reward is the positive outcome or benefit you experience after completing the routine. It reinforces the behavior, making it more likely to be repeated in the future. Rewards can be tangible, like enjoying a piece of dark chocolate after a workout, or intangible, such as experiencing a sense of accomplishment or relaxation. The reward creates a positive association with the routine, strengthening the habit loop. Identifying meaningful rewards can motivate you to stick with your new habits.

Consistency and Repetition Consistency and repetition are fundamental to solidifying new habits. It's essential to perform the desired behavior regularly and consistently, even when motivation wanes. Research suggests that it takes, on average, 66 days to form a new habit, although this can vary depending on the complexity of the behavior and individual differences. Developing a routine that fits seamlessly into your daily life can help you stay consistent. For instance, if you aim to incorporate a daily exercise habit, choose a specific time each day that works best for you and stick to it.

Breaking Unhealthy Habits Understanding the habit loop also provides insights into how to break unhealthy habits. By identifying the cues and rewards associated with an undesirable behavior, you can disrupt the habit loop and replace the routine with a healthier alternative. For example, if stress triggers you to eat unhealthy snacks, recognize the cue (stress) and reward (temporary relief) and replace the routine with a healthier stress-relief activity, such as taking a walk, practicing deep breathing, or engaging in a hobby.

Implementation Intentions Creating implementation intentions is a powerful strategy to support habit formation. This involves planning out specific actions you will take in response to particular cues. An implementation intention typically follows the structure: "If [cue], then I will [routine]." For example, "If it's 6 AM, then I will go for a 30-minute run." By clearly defining when and where you will perform the behavior, you increase the likelihood of following through.

Self-Reflection and Adaptation Regular self-reflection and adaptation are essential for habit formation. Periodically assess your progress, identify any challenges or barriers, and make necessary adjustments. Celebrate small wins and milestones to maintain motivation and reinforce positive behavior. Be patient with yourself and recognize that setbacks are a natural part of the process. Learn from them and continue working towards your goals.

In conclusion, understanding the psychology of habit formation is crucial for building and maintaining healthy habits. By recognizing the habit loop, focusing on consistency and repetition, and employing strategies like implementation intentions and self-reflection, you can create lasting positive changes in your life. Embrace the journey of habit formation and leverage the power of psychology to achieve your health and wellness goals.

Setting Realistic and Achievable Goals

Setting realistic and achievable goals is a cornerstone of building healthy habits. Goals provide direction, motivation, and a sense of purpose, helping you stay focused and committed to positive changes. To be effective, goals should be clearly defined, manageable, and aligned with your overall wellness objectives. Here's how to set and achieve realistic goals using the SMART framework.

Specific: Clearly Define Your Goals Specific goals are clear and detailed, answering the who, what, where, when, and why of your objective. Instead of setting a vague goal like "exercise more," specify what type of exercise you will do, how often, and for how long. For example, "I will go for a 30-minute jog every Monday, Wednesday, and Friday after work." Clear goals provide a concrete plan and make it easier to track progress.

Measurable: Track Your Progress Measurable goals allow you to quantify your progress and determine when you have achieved your objective. Include metrics such as duration, frequency, or quantity in your goals. For instance, if your goal is to drink more water, specify the amount, such as "I will drink eight 8-ounce glasses of water each day." Tracking your progress helps you stay motivated and provides a sense of accomplishment as you see your improvements over time.

Achievable: Set Realistic Expectations Achievable goals are realistic and attainable within your current capabilities and resources. Setting overly ambitious goals can lead to frustration and discouragement if they are not met. Assess your starting point and consider any potential obstacles when setting your goals. For example, if you're new to running, it's more realistic to start with a goal of jogging for 10 minutes a day and gradually increasing the duration, rather than aiming to run a marathon right away. Breaking down larger goals into smaller, manageable steps makes them more achievable and helps build confidence.

Relevant: Align Goals with Your Priorities Relevant goals are meaningful and aligned with your broader health and wellness priorities. Consider why the goal is important to you and how it fits into your overall vision for a healthier lifestyle. For example, if improving your cardiovascular health is a priority, setting a goal to engage in regular aerobic exercise, such as cycling or swimming, is relevant. Ensuring your goals are aligned with your values and long-term objectives increases your commitment and motivation to achieve them.

Time-bound: Set a Timeline Time-bound goals have a specific deadline or timeframe, providing a sense of urgency and helping you stay focused. Establishing a clear timeline encourages consistent effort and prevents procrastination. For example, "I will lose 10 pounds in three months" sets a specific timeframe for achieving your weight loss goal. Break down the timeframe into smaller milestones to maintain momentum and celebrate progress along the way.

Breaking Down Goals into Manageable Steps Large goals can sometimes feel overwhelming, making it challenging to know where to start. Breaking down your goals into smaller, manageable steps makes them more approachable and less daunting. For example, if your goal is to adopt a healthier diet, start with specific actions such as incorporating one additional serving of vegetables into your meals each day or preparing homemade lunches three times a week. As you achieve these smaller steps, gradually build on them to work towards your larger goal.

Staying Motivated and Tracking Progress Maintaining motivation is key to achieving your goals. Celebrate small wins and milestones to acknowledge your progress and reinforce positive behavior. Keeping a journal or using a tracking app can help you monitor your progress and stay accountable. Reflect on your achievements regularly and adjust your goals as needed to stay challenged and motivated.

In conclusion, setting realistic and achievable goals using the SMART framework is essential for building healthy habits. By defining specific, measurable, achievable, relevant, and time-bound goals, you can create a clear plan of action and stay focused on your wellness journey. Break down larger goals into manageable steps, track your progress, and celebrate your achievements along the way. Embrace the power of goal-setting as a tool for positive change and enjoy the rewards of a healthier lifestyle.

Creating a Supportive Environment

The environment in which we live and work has a profound impact on our ability to build and maintain healthy habits. By creating a supportive environment, you can enhance your chances of success and make it easier to adopt and sustain positive behaviors. This involves organizing your physical space, surrounding yourself with supportive people, and reducing exposure to triggers of unhealthy behaviors. Here's how to create an environment that fosters healthy habits.

Organizing Your Space The physical environment plays a significant role in shaping our behaviors. A cluttered, disorganized space can lead to stress, distractions, and difficulty in sticking to healthy habits. Start by organizing your living and working spaces to make healthy choices more accessible and convenient. Here are some tips to get started:

Kitchen: Keep healthy foods, such as fruits, vegetables, and whole grains, easily accessible. Arrange your pantry and refrigerator to highlight nutritious options and keep unhealthy snacks out of sight. Prepare healthy meals and snacks in advance, so they are readily available when you're hungry.

Workspace: Create a clutter-free and ergonomic workspace that promotes productivity and well-being. Keep water nearby to stay hydrated, and take regular breaks to stretch and move around. Consider adding plants or natural elements to your workspace to reduce stress and enhance focus.

Exercise Area: Designate a specific area in your home for physical activity, whether it's a corner for yoga or space for home workouts. Keep exercise equipment, such as dumbbells, resistance bands, or a yoga mat, within easy reach to encourage regular use.

Surrounding Yourself with Supportive People The social environment is equally important in supporting healthy habits. Surrounding yourself with people who encourage and motivate you can make a significant difference in your success. Here are some strategies to build a supportive social network:

Family and Friends: Communicate your goals and intentions to your family and friends. Let them know how they can support you and ask for their encouragement. Engage in healthy activities together, such as cooking nutritious meals or exercising as a group.

Community Groups: Join community groups or clubs that share your interests and goals. Whether it's a fitness class, a hiking group, or a cooking club, being part of a community provides accountability, motivation, and a sense of belonging.

Online Communities: If in-person groups are not accessible, consider joining online communities or forums related to your goals. Online platforms can offer valuable support, advice, and inspiration from people who share similar experiences and challenges.

Reducing Exposure to Triggers Identifying and reducing exposure to triggers of unhealthy behaviors is crucial for creating a supportive environment. Triggers can be anything that prompts you to engage in behaviors you're trying to change, such as stress, boredom, or specific environments. Here are some strategies to minimize exposure to triggers:

Stress Management: Develop healthy coping mechanisms for stress, such as meditation, deep breathing exercises, or engaging in hobbies. Avoid using unhealthy habits, such as smoking or overeating, as stress relievers.

Healthy Alternatives: Replace triggers with healthy alternatives. For example, if you tend to snack mindlessly while watching TV, swap unhealthy snacks for nutritious options like fruit or nuts. If boredom is a trigger, find engaging activities that keep you occupied, such as reading, crafting, or exercising.

Environmental Cues: Modify your environment to remove or reduce cues that trigger unhealthy behaviors. For instance, if you're trying to reduce screen time, set up a designated charging station for your devices outside of your bedroom. If you're aiming to eat healthier, avoid keeping junk food in the house.

Creating Accountability: Accountability is a powerful tool for maintaining healthy habits. Sharing your goals with others and regularly checking in on your progress can help you stay committed and motivated. Here are some ways to create accountability:

Accountability Partners: Find an accountability partner who shares similar goals and can provide mutual support and motivation. Regularly check in with each other, share progress, and celebrate achievements.

Tracking Progress: Use tools such as journals, apps, or calendars to track your progress and stay accountable to yourself. Monitoring your progress provides a sense of accomplishment and helps identify areas for improvement.

Professional Support: Seek support from professionals, such as a nutritionist, personal trainer, or therapist, who can provide guidance, accountability, and expertise. Regular appointments and check-ins with professionals can help you stay on track and address any challenges.

In conclusion, creating a supportive environment is essential for building and maintaining healthy habits. By organizing your physical space, surrounding yourself with supportive people, reducing exposure to triggers, and creating accountability, you can enhance your chances of success and make healthy choices more accessible and sustainable. Embrace these strategies to foster a positive environment that supports your wellness journey and enjoy the benefits of a healthier lifestyle.

Overcoming Barriers and Staying Motivated

Building and maintaining healthy habits can be challenging, especially when faced with common barriers such as lack of time, motivation, and resources. However, by identifying these obstacles and implementing effective strategies, you can overcome them and stay on track with your wellness goals. Here's how to tackle these challenges and maintain motivation on your journey to a healthier lifestyle.

Time Management One of the most common barriers to building healthy habits is the perception of having no time. Busy work schedules, family obligations, and other responsibilities can make it seem impossible to fit in healthy activities. However, effective time management can help you carve out time for your wellness goals. Start by prioritizing your health and recognizing that taking care of yourself is essential for overall well-being. Here are some strategies to manage your time effectively:

Schedule Your Activities: Treat your healthy habits as non-negotiable appointments. Block out specific times in your calendar for exercise, meal preparation, and self-care activities. Consistency is key, so try to stick to your schedule as closely as possible.

Break Tasks into Smaller Steps: Instead of trying to fit in a long workout session, break it into shorter, more manageable chunks. For example, if you can't find an hour for exercise, try three 20-minute sessions throughout the day. Similarly, break down meal preparation into smaller tasks, such as chopping vegetables in advance or cooking in bulk on weekends.

Multitask Wisely: Combine activities to make the most of your time. For instance, you can listen to an audiobook or a podcast while exercising or do stretches while watching TV. Find creative ways to integrate healthy habits into your daily routine without adding extra time.

Finding Intrinsic Motivation Intrinsic motivation, or the internal drive to engage in a behavior for its own sake, is more sustainable than external motivation, which relies on external rewards or pressures. Identifying your intrinsic motivation can help you stay committed to your health goals. Reflect on why you want to build healthy habits and how they align with your values and long-term aspirations. Here are some tips to find and maintain intrinsic motivation:

Connect with Your Why: Identify the deeper reasons behind your health goals. For example, you might want to improve your fitness to feel more energetic, reduce stress, or set a positive example for your children. Keep these reasons in mind when you face challenges or setbacks.

Focus on Enjoyment: Choose activities that you genuinely enjoy and look forward to. If you love dancing, take a dance class instead of forcing yourself to do an exercise you dislike. Finding joy in the process makes it easier to stick with healthy habits.

Celebrate Small Wins: Recognize and celebrate your progress, no matter how small. Each step forward is an achievement that brings you closer to your goals. Celebrating small wins boosts your confidence and reinforces positive behavior.

Seeking Support Having a support system can make a significant difference in overcoming barriers and staying motivated. Surround yourself with people who encourage and support your wellness journey. Here's how to build a strong support network:

Share Your Goals: Communicate your health goals with family and friends. Let them know how they can support you and ask for their encouragement. Having someone to share your progress and challenges with can provide accountability and motivation.

Join Support Groups: Consider joining support groups or communities, either in-person or online, that share similar goals. Support groups offer a platform to share experiences, gain insights, and receive encouragement from others who understand your journey.

Professional Guidance: Seek support from professionals, such as a personal trainer, nutritionist, or therapist, who can provide expert guidance and personalized advice. Regular check-ins with professionals can help you stay on track and address any challenges that arise.

Maintaining a Positive Mindset A positive mindset is essential for overcoming barriers and staying motivated. Cultivate a growth mindset, which involves viewing challenges as opportunities for growth and learning. Here are some strategies to maintain a positive outlook:

Practice Self-Compassion: Be kind to yourself and recognize that setbacks are a natural part of the journey. Instead of being self-critical, focus on what you can learn from the experience and how you can improve moving forward.

Visualize Success: Use visualization techniques to imagine yourself achieving your goals and enjoying the benefits of your healthy habits. Visualization can boost motivation and reinforce your commitment to your goals.

Surround Yourself with Positivity: Engage in activities and surround yourself with people who uplift and inspire you. Positive influences can help you stay focused and motivated on your wellness journey.

In conclusion, overcoming barriers and staying motivated requires effective time management, intrinsic motivation, a strong support system, and a positive mindset. By implementing these strategies, you can tackle challenges, maintain healthy habits, and achieve your wellness goals. Embrace the journey with determination and enjoy the rewards of a healthier, more fulfilling lifestyle.

Long-Term Maintenance and Adaptation

Building healthy habits is an ongoing process that requires long-term maintenance and the ability to adapt to changing circumstances. Sustaining these habits over time is essential for achieving lasting health benefits and overall well-being. Here's how to integrate healthy habits into your lifestyle permanently and remain flexible in adjusting them as needed.

Integrating Habits into Your Lifestyle To ensure that healthy habits become a permanent part of your life, it's important to integrate them seamlessly into your daily routine. Consistency is key to maintaining these habits over the long term. Here are some strategies to help you embed healthy behaviors into your lifestyle:

Routine and Structure: Establishing a daily routine that includes your healthy habits can help make them second nature. For example, if exercise is a priority, schedule it at the same time each day, such as a morning workout or an evening walk after dinner. Consistent routines reduce the likelihood of skipping important activities and make it easier to stick with your habits.

Habits Stacking: Habit stacking involves linking a new habit to an existing one, creating a chain of behaviors that support each other. For example, if you want to build a habit of stretching, do it immediately after brushing your teeth in the morning. By associating the new habit with an established one, you reinforce the behavior and make it more automatic.

Simplify and Automate: Simplify your environment to make healthy choices more accessible and reduce decision fatigue. Prepare healthy meals in advance, keep exercise equipment within reach, and set up reminders or alarms for important activities. Automating certain tasks, such as setting up automatic deliveries for healthy groceries, can also help maintain consistency.

Adaptability and Flexibility Life is dynamic, and circumstances can change, requiring you to adapt your habits accordingly. Flexibility is crucial for maintaining healthy behaviors over the long term. Here's how to stay adaptable and resilient:

Adjusting Goals: Regularly reassess your goals and adjust them as needed to reflect changes in your life, such as new responsibilities, health conditions, or personal preferences. Be open to modifying your goals to stay aligned with your current situation. For example, if you experience a busy period at work, adjust your exercise routine to shorter, more frequent sessions rather than longer ones.

Embrace Setbacks: Recognize that setbacks are a natural part of the journey. Instead of viewing them as failures, treat them as opportunities to learn and grow. Reflect on what led to the setback and identify strategies to overcome similar challenges in the future. Embrace a growth mindset, which involves seeing challenges as chances to develop and improve.

Stay Mindful: Practice mindfulness to stay attuned to your body and mind. Mindfulness helps you recognize when certain habits need adjustment and allows you to respond proactively. For example, if you notice increased stress, incorporate additional relaxation techniques or adjust your schedule to allow for more rest.

Regular Self-Reflection: Self-reflection is a powerful tool for sustaining healthy habits and making necessary adjustments. Periodically assess your progress, identify areas for improvement, and celebrate your achievements. Here are some self-reflection practices to consider:

Journaling: Keep a journal to document your journey, track your progress, and reflect on your experiences. Write about your successes, challenges, and any insights gained along the way. Journaling provides a space for self-expression and helps reinforce positive behaviors.

Set Milestones: Establish milestones to mark significant progress and celebrate your achievements. Milestones provide motivation and a sense of accomplishment, reinforcing your commitment to healthy habits.

Seek Feedback: Ask for feedback from trusted friends, family, or professionals who can offer valuable perspectives on your progress. Constructive feedback can help you identify blind spots and areas for improvement.

Maintaining Motivation Sustaining healthy habits over the long term requires ongoing motivation. Here are some strategies to keep your motivation high:

Variety and Fun: Introduce variety into your routines to prevent boredom and keep things interesting. Try new activities, recipes, or challenges to keep yourself engaged and motivated. Enjoyment is key to long-term adherence.

Positive Reinforcement: Use positive reinforcement to reward yourself for sticking to your habits. Rewards can be simple, such as treating yourself to a relaxing bath, enjoying a favorite hobby, or spending time with loved ones. Positive reinforcement reinforces the behavior and makes it more likely to continue.

Inspire Others: Sharing your journey and inspiring others can boost your motivation. By setting a positive example and encouraging others to adopt healthy habits, you reinforce your own commitment and create a supportive community.

In conclusion, long-term maintenance and adaptation are essential for sustaining healthy habits and achieving lasting health benefits. By integrating habits into your lifestyle, remaining flexible and adaptable, practicing regular self-reflection, and maintaining motivation, you can enjoy the rewards of a healthier, more fulfilling life. Embrace the journey of continuous improvement and stay committed to your wellness goals, no matter what life brings your way.

Chapter 9: Emotional Well-being

Understanding Emotional Well-being

Summary: Define emotional well-being and its significance in overall health. Discuss the components of emotional well-being, including self-awareness, emotional regulation, and resilience. Explain how emotional well-being impacts relationships, decision-making, and physical health. Highlight the importance of recognizing and addressing emotions.

Developing Self-Awareness

Summary: Explore the concept of self-awareness and its role in emotional well-being. Discuss techniques for increasing self-awareness, such as mindfulness, journaling, and self-reflection. Emphasize the importance of understanding personal triggers, strengths, and areas for growth. Provide practical exercises for enhancing self-awareness.

Emotional Regulation and Coping Strategies

Summary: Discuss the importance of emotional regulation in maintaining emotional well-being. Outline various coping strategies for managing emotions, including deep breathing, cognitive reframing, and physical activity. Highlight the role of therapy and counseling in developing effective emotional regulation skills. Provide tips for creating a personalized coping toolkit.

Building Resilience

Summary: Define resilience and its significance in emotional well-being. Explore strategies for building resilience, such as fostering a positive mindset, developing problem-solving skills, and seeking social support. Discuss the role of adversity in strengthening resilience and how to use challenges as opportunities for growth. Provide examples of resilient behaviors and mindsets.

Nurturing Positive Relationships

Summary: Examine the impact of relationships on emotional well-being. Discuss the characteristics of healthy relationships and the importance of communication, empathy, and trust. Provide strategies for building and maintaining positive relationships, including setting boundaries, practicing active listening, and showing appreciation. Highlight the benefits of social connections and the role of community in emotional health.

This outline covers the essential aspects of emotional well-being, focusing on understanding emotions, developing self-awareness, regulating emotions, building resilience, and nurturing positive relationships. Ready to dive into writing any of these points, or something else in mind?

Emotional well-being is a vital component of overall health, encompassing our ability to understand, manage, and express our emotions effectively. It involves a state of balance where individuals can cope with life's challenges, build meaningful relationships, and maintain a positive outlook. Recognizing and nurturing emotional well-being is essential for leading a fulfilling and resilient life.

Defining Emotional Well-being Emotional well-being is the ability to experience, recognize, and manage a wide range of emotions, from joy and contentment to sadness and frustration. It is not about being happy all the time but rather about having the skills to navigate through different emotional states healthily and constructively. Emotional well-being includes several key components:

Self-awareness: Understanding your emotions, triggers, and how they affect your thoughts and behaviors.

Emotional regulation: The ability to manage and respond to emotions appropriately, without being overwhelmed by them.

Resilience: The capacity to bounce back from adversity, stress, and challenges with a positive mindset.

Social connections: Building and maintaining healthy relationships that provide support, empathy, and a sense of belonging.

The Impact of Emotional Well-being on Overall Health Emotional well-being has a profound impact on various aspects of our lives, influencing our physical health, relationships, decision-making, and overall quality of life. Here's how emotional well-being affects different areas:

Physical Health: Emotions and physical health are closely linked. Chronic stress, anxiety, and negative emotions can lead to physical health issues such as headaches, digestive problems, high blood pressure, and weakened immune function. On the other hand, positive emotions and effective emotional management can promote better health outcomes, reduce the risk of chronic diseases, and enhance overall well-being.

Relationships: Emotional well-being plays a crucial role in building and maintaining healthy relationships. Self-awareness and emotional regulation enable individuals to communicate effectively, resolve conflicts, and empathize with others. Healthy relationships provide emotional support, reduce feelings of loneliness, and contribute to a sense of belonging and happiness.

Decision-making: Emotions influence our decision-making processes. When we are in a positive emotional state, we are more likely to make thoughtful and rational decisions. Conversely, negative emotions such as anger or fear can cloud judgment and lead to impulsive or irrational choices. Emotional well-being helps individuals make informed decisions that align with their values and long-term goals.

Quality of Life: A balanced emotional state contributes to a higher quality of life. Individuals with good emotional well-being tend to experience greater life satisfaction, purpose, and fulfillment. They are better equipped to handle life's challenges, adapt to changes, and pursue their passions and interests.

Recognizing and Addressing Emotions Understanding and acknowledging emotions is the first step toward emotional well-being. It's essential to recognize that all emotions, whether positive or negative, serve a purpose and provide valuable information about our experiences and needs. Here are some strategies for recognizing and addressing emotions:

Mindfulness: Practicing mindfulness involves paying attention to the present moment without judgment. Mindfulness helps individuals become aware of their emotions and thoughts, allowing them to respond rather than react impulsively. Mindfulness techniques, such as meditation and deep breathing, can enhance emotional awareness and regulation.

Journaling: Writing down your thoughts and feelings can provide clarity and insight into your emotional state. Journaling allows you to explore and process emotions, identify patterns and triggers, and develop a deeper understanding of yourself.

Emotional Expression: Expressing emotions in healthy ways, such as talking to a trusted friend, engaging in creative activities, or practicing physical activities, can help release emotional tension and promote well-being. It's important to find outlets that allow you to express and process emotions constructively.

Seeking Support: Reaching out for support from friends, family, or mental health professionals can provide valuable perspective and guidance. Sharing your emotions and experiences with others can alleviate feelings of isolation and help you navigate challenges more effectively.

In conclusion, emotional well-being is a fundamental aspect of overall health that influences various areas of our lives. By understanding the components of emotional well-being, recognizing the impact of emotions, and adopting strategies to manage and express emotions constructively, individuals can enhance their quality of life and build resilience. Embrace the journey of emotional well-being and prioritize it as an essential part of your health and wellness goals.

Developing Self-Awareness

Self-awareness is the foundation of emotional well-being. It involves understanding your emotions, thoughts, and behaviors and recognizing how they influence your interactions and decisions. Developing self-awareness allows you to navigate life's challenges more effectively, build stronger relationships, and achieve a deeper sense of fulfillment. Here's how to enhance self-awareness and its importance in emotional well-being.

The Role of Self-Awareness: Self-awareness is the ability to introspect and reflect on your inner experiences. It enables you to identify your strengths, weaknesses, values, and goals. By understanding your emotional triggers and patterns, you can respond to situations more thoughtfully rather than reacting impulsively. Self-awareness also fosters emotional intelligence, which is crucial for building empathy, improving communication, and managing conflicts.

Mindfulness Practices Mindfulness is a powerful tool for developing self-awareness. It involves paying attention to the present moment without judgment, allowing you to observe your thoughts and feelings with clarity. Here are some mindfulness practices to enhance self-awareness:

Meditation: Set aside a few minutes each day for meditation. Find a quiet space, sit comfortably, and focus on your breath. Observe your thoughts and emotions as they arise without trying to change or judge them. Meditation helps you become more aware of your mental and emotional states, promoting a sense of calm and insight.

Body Scan: A body scan involves paying attention to physical sensations throughout your body. Lie down or sit comfortably and slowly move your focus from your toes to your head, noticing any areas of tension or discomfort. This practice helps you connect with your body and become more attuned to your physical and emotional well-being.

Mindful Breathing: Practice mindful breathing by taking slow, deep breaths and paying attention to the sensations of each inhale and exhale. This technique can be done anywhere and helps anchor you in the present moment, enhancing your awareness of your thoughts and feelings.

Journaling: Journaling is an effective way to explore and process your emotions. Writing down your thoughts and feelings allows you to reflect on your experiences and gain insights into your emotional patterns. Here are some journaling prompts to enhance self-awareness:

Daily Reflection: At the end of each day, write about your experiences, emotions, and any challenges you faced. Reflect on how you responded to situations and what you learned from them.

Emotion Exploration: Choose an emotion you felt strongly during the day and explore it in your journal. Describe the circumstances that triggered it, how you felt physically and mentally, and how you responded. Reflect on what this emotion tells you about your needs and values.

Gratitude Journaling: Write about the things you are grateful for each day. Focusing on positive experiences and appreciation can enhance your emotional well-being and shift your perspective.

Self-Reflection Regular self-reflection helps you gain deeper insights into your thoughts, feelings, and behaviors. Set aside time for self-reflection and consider the following exercises:

Strengths and Weaknesses: Identify your strengths and weaknesses. Reflect on how you can leverage your strengths and work on areas for improvement. Understanding your capabilities and limitations helps you set realistic goals and develop a growth mindset.

Values and Goals: Clarify your core values and long-term goals. Reflect on how your daily actions align with these values and goals. Identifying any discrepancies can help you make necessary adjustments to live more authentically and purposefully.

Trigger Analysis: Reflect on situations that triggered strong emotional reactions. Analyze what specifically triggered you, why it affected you, and how you can respond differently in the future. Understanding your triggers helps you manage your emotions more effectively.

Feedback and Perspective Seeking feedback from others provides valuable insights into how your behavior is perceived and how it impacts your relationships. Here are some tips for seeking feedback:

Ask Trusted Individuals: Reach out to friends, family, or colleagues whom you trust and respect. Ask for honest feedback about your strengths and areas for improvement. Be open to their perspectives and consider how you can use the feedback for personal growth.

Professional Support: Consider working with a therapist or coach who can provide objective feedback and guidance. Professionals can help you explore your emotions, develop self-awareness, and implement strategies for personal development.

Personal Growth and Adaptation Developing self-awareness is an ongoing process that requires continuous effort and adaptation. Here are some practices to support your personal growth:

Set Intentions: Set clear intentions for your self-awareness journey. Identify specific areas you want to focus on and create actionable steps to achieve your goals.

Practice Patience: Developing self-awareness takes time and patience. Be kind to yourself and recognize that growth is a gradual process. Celebrate small milestones and progress along the way.

Stay Curious: Cultivate a mindset of curiosity and openness. Embrace new experiences and challenges as opportunities to learn more about yourself. Curiosity fosters self-discovery and enhances emotional well-being.

In conclusion, developing self-awareness is a fundamental aspect of emotional well-being that empowers you to understand and manage your emotions effectively. By practicing mindfulness, journaling, self-reflection, seeking feedback, and embracing personal growth, you can enhance your self-awareness and navigate life's challenges with greater resilience and insight. Embrace the journey of self-discovery and prioritize self-awareness as an essential part of your emotional well-being.

Emotional Regulation and Coping Strategies

Emotional regulation is the ability to manage and respond to emotional experiences in a healthy and balanced way. It is a crucial aspect of emotional well-being, enabling individuals to navigate life's challenges with resilience and stability. Effective emotional regulation involves recognizing, understanding, and appropriately expressing emotions. Here's a deeper dive into the importance of emotional regulation and various coping strategies to support it.

The Importance of Emotional Regulation Emotional regulation is essential for maintaining mental health and overall well-being. It allows individuals to cope with stress, build strong relationships, and make thoughtful decisions. Without proper emotional regulation, emotions can become overwhelming and lead to negative outcomes such as anxiety, depression, and impulsive behaviors. Developing skills for managing emotions can improve quality of life and enhance emotional resilience.

Coping Strategies for Emotional Regulation There are various coping strategies that can help individuals manage their emotions effectively. Here are some techniques to support emotional regulation:

Deep Breathing: Deep breathing exercises can help calm the nervous system and reduce stress. Practice taking slow, deep breaths, inhaling through your nose, and exhaling through your mouth. Focus on the sensation of the breath entering and leaving your body. This technique can be done anywhere and helps to center your mind and body.

Cognitive Reframing: Cognitive reframing involves changing the way you think about a situation to alter its emotional impact. Instead of focusing on negative aspects, try to find a positive or neutral perspective. For example, if you are feeling stressed about a work deadline, reframe it as an opportunity to showcase your skills and work efficiently. This shift in thinking can help reduce negative emotions and promote a more balanced outlook.

Physical Activity: Engaging in physical activity is a powerful way to regulate emotions. Exercise releases endorphins, which are natural mood elevators. Whether it's a brisk walk, yoga, or a high-intensity workout, physical activity can help reduce stress, anxiety, and depression. Find activities that you enjoy and make them a regular part of your routine.

Mindfulness and Meditation: Mindfulness and meditation practices can enhance emotional regulation by promoting awareness and acceptance of emotions. Mindfulness involves paying attention to the present moment without judgment. Meditation techniques, such as loving-kindness meditation or body scan meditation, can help you connect with your emotions and develop a compassionate attitude towards yourself.

Creative Expression: Engaging in creative activities, such as painting, writing, or playing music, can provide an outlet for expressing and processing emotions. Creative expression allows you to channel your feelings into a tangible form, helping you gain insight and release emotional tension.

Social Support: Talking to a trusted friend, family member, or therapist can provide valuable support and perspective. Sharing your emotions with others can help you feel understood and less isolated. Social connections play a significant role in emotional regulation, offering comfort and encouragement during challenging times.

Therapy and Counseling Therapy and counseling can be invaluable resources for developing emotional regulation skills. Cognitive-behavioral therapy (CBT) is a widely used approach that helps individuals identify and change negative thought patterns and behaviors. Through CBT, individuals can learn effective coping strategies and develop healthier ways of responding to emotions.

Dialectical behavior therapy (DBT) is another therapeutic approach that focuses on emotional regulation, distress tolerance, and interpersonal effectiveness. DBT teaches skills for managing intense emotions, improving relationships, and reducing self-destructive behaviors. Seeking professional support can provide personalized guidance and help you build a toolkit of coping strategies tailored to your needs.

Creating a Personalized Coping Toolkit Building a personalized coping toolkit involves identifying and practicing coping strategies that work best for you. Here are some steps to create your own toolkit:

Identify Triggers: Reflect on situations or experiences that tend to trigger strong emotional reactions. Understanding your triggers helps you anticipate and prepare for them.

Choose Strategies: Experiment with different coping strategies to find what works best for you. Select a variety of techniques that address different aspects of emotional regulation, such as physical activity, mindfulness, and social support.

Practice Regularly: Incorporate coping strategies into your daily routine to build and reinforce your skills. Consistent practice helps make these techniques more effective and accessible when you need them.

Evaluate and Adjust: Regularly assess the effectiveness of your coping toolkit. If certain strategies are not working, be open to trying new ones. Adjust your toolkit as needed to ensure it remains relevant and supportive.

Embracing Emotional Regulation Emotional regulation is an ongoing process that requires self-awareness, practice, and commitment. By developing and utilizing coping strategies, you can enhance your emotional well-being and navigate life's challenges with greater ease. Embrace the journey of emotional regulation, and prioritize your emotional health as a key aspect of your overall well-being.

In conclusion, emotional regulation is essential for maintaining mental health and overall well-being. By adopting coping strategies such as deep breathing, cognitive reframing, physical activity, mindfulness, creative expression, and seeking social support, you can effectively manage your emotions and enhance your emotional resilience. Creating a personalized coping toolkit and seeking professional support through therapy and counseling can further support your emotional regulation journey. Embrace these strategies to build a balanced and fulfilling life.

Building Resilience

Resilience is the ability to bounce back from adversity, stress, and challenges with strength and optimism. It's a crucial component of emotional well-being, enabling individuals to navigate difficult situations and emerge stronger. Building resilience involves developing a positive mindset, problem-solving skills, and seeking social support. Here's how to cultivate resilience and use challenges as opportunities for growth.

Defining Resilience: Resilience is not about avoiding adversity but rather about adapting to and recovering from it. It's the capacity to maintain or regain emotional equilibrium in the face of stress, trauma, or setbacks. Resilient individuals can cope with challenges, learn from experiences, and continue moving forward. Resilience is a dynamic process that can be developed and strengthened over time.

Fostering a Positive Mindset A positive mindset is fundamental to building resilience. It involves viewing challenges as opportunities for growth rather than as insurmountable obstacles. Here are some strategies to foster a positive mindset:

Embrace Optimism: Practice looking for the silver lining in difficult situations. Focus on what you can learn from the experience and how it can contribute to your personal growth. Optimism doesn't mean ignoring problems but rather approaching them with a hopeful and solution-oriented attitude.

Gratitude Practice: Cultivate gratitude by regularly reflecting on the positive aspects of your life. Keeping a gratitude journal and noting down things you are thankful for each day can shift your focus from what's wrong to what's going well. Gratitude fosters a positive outlook and enhances emotional well-being.

Self-Compassion: Be kind to yourself and recognize that everyone faces challenges. Treat yourself with the same compassion and understanding that you would offer to a friend. Self-compassion helps you manage setbacks without self-criticism and promotes emotional resilience.

Developing Problem-Solving Skills Effective problem-solving skills are essential for resilience. They enable you to identify challenges, generate solutions, and take action. Here's how to enhance your problem-solving abilities:

Identify the Problem: Clearly define the problem or challenge you are facing. Break it down into manageable parts to understand its components and underlying causes.

Generate Solutions: Brainstorm multiple potential solutions to the problem. Consider both short-term and long-term strategies. Don't be afraid to think outside the box and explore creative options.

Evaluate and Choose: Assess the pros and cons of each potential solution. Consider the feasibility, resources required, and potential outcomes. Choose the solution that best addresses the problem and aligns with your goals.

Take Action: Implement the chosen solution with confidence. Monitor the progress and be willing to make adjustments as needed. Taking proactive steps empowers you to manage challenges effectively.

Seeking Social Support Social support plays a significant role in building resilience. Strong relationships provide emotional comfort, practical assistance, and a sense of belonging. Here's how to cultivate and utilize social support:

Build Connections: Nurture your relationships with family, friends, and colleagues. Make an effort to spend quality time with loved ones and engage in meaningful conversations. Building strong connections creates a support network you can rely on during difficult times.

Seek Help: Don't hesitate to reach out for support when needed. Sharing your experiences and emotions with trusted individuals can provide relief and perspective. Whether it's talking to a friend, joining a support group, or seeking professional counseling, seeking help is a sign of strength.

Offer Support: Providing support to others can also enhance your resilience. Acts of kindness, empathy, and compassion towards others foster a sense of community and reinforce positive social connections.

Using Challenges as Opportunities for Growth Adversity can be a powerful teacher, offering valuable lessons and opportunities for growth. Here's how to use challenges to build resilience:

Reflect and Learn: After facing a difficult situation, take time to reflect on the experience. Consider what you learned about yourself, your strengths, and areas for improvement. Reflection helps you gain insight and develop a growth mindset.

Adapt and Grow: Use the lessons learned from adversity to make positive changes in your life. Adapt your strategies, set new goals, and continue striving for personal growth. Embrace the idea that challenges can lead to transformation and development.

Maintain Perspective: Keep a long-term perspective on challenges. Recognize that difficulties are often temporary and that you have the capacity to overcome them. Maintaining perspective helps you stay focused on your goals and maintain resilience.

In conclusion, building resilience is essential for emotional well-being and navigating life's challenges with strength and optimism. By fostering a positive mindset, developing problem-solving skills, seeking social support, and using challenges as opportunities for growth, you can enhance your resilience and thrive in the face of adversity. Embrace resilience as a dynamic process and continue to cultivate it as part of your emotional well-being journey.

Nurturing Positive Relationships

Positive relationships are a cornerstone of emotional well-being. They provide support, joy, and a sense of belonging. Cultivating and maintaining healthy relationships requires effort, communication, and empathy. By nurturing positive connections, individuals can enhance their emotional health and overall quality of life. Here's how to build and sustain meaningful relationships.

The Impact of Relationships on Emotional Well-being Healthy relationships have a profound impact on emotional well-being. They offer emotional support, reduce feelings of loneliness, and create a sense of security and belonging. Positive relationships contribute to increased life satisfaction, reduced stress, and improved mental health. Conversely, toxic or strained relationships can lead to stress, anxiety, and emotional distress. Understanding the importance of relationships and prioritizing their quality is essential for emotional well-being.

Characteristics of Healthy Relationships Healthy relationships are built on a foundation of trust, respect, and mutual understanding. Here are some key characteristics of positive relationships:

Trust: Trust is the cornerstone of any healthy relationship. It involves having confidence in the other person's integrity and reliability. Trust is built through consistent honesty, transparency, and dependability.

Respect: Respect involves valuing each other's opinions, boundaries, and individuality. It means treating each other with kindness and consideration, even during disagreements.

Communication: Effective communication is essential for understanding and connecting with others. It involves active listening, expressing thoughts and feelings clearly, and being open to feedback. Good communication fosters intimacy and prevents misunderstandings.

Empathy: Empathy is the ability to understand and share the feelings of others. It involves putting yourself in the other person's shoes and responding with compassion. Empathy strengthens connections and enhances emotional support.

Mutual Support: In healthy relationships, individuals support each other's goals, dreams, and well-being. They offer encouragement, celebrate successes, and provide comfort during challenging times. Mutual support fosters a sense of partnership and collaboration.

Strategies for Building Positive Relationships Building and maintaining positive relationships requires intentional effort and commitment. Here are some strategies to nurture healthy connections:

Set Boundaries: Establishing and respecting boundaries is essential for maintaining healthy relationships. Boundaries define what is acceptable and what is not, helping to protect your emotional and mental well-being. Communicate your boundaries clearly and respectfully, and be open to hearing and respecting others' boundaries.

Practice Active Listening: Active listening involves fully engaging with the other person, paying attention to their words, and responding thoughtfully. Avoid interrupting or planning your response while the other person is speaking. Show that you are listening through verbal affirmations, nodding, and maintaining eye contact. Active listening fosters understanding and connection.

Show Appreciation: Expressing gratitude and appreciation strengthens relationships and fosters positive feelings. Acknowledge and appreciate the efforts, qualities, and contributions of others. Small gestures of kindness, such as saying thank you or offering compliments, can make a significant impact.

Be Present: Being present means giving your full attention to the other person during interactions. Put away distractions, such as phones or electronic devices, and focus on the conversation. Being present shows that you value and prioritize the relationship.

Resolve Conflicts Constructively: Conflicts are a natural part of any relationship, but how they are handled determines their impact. Approach conflicts with a calm and open mindset. Use "I" statements to express your feelings and avoid blaming or criticizing the other person. Seek to understand their perspective and work together to find a resolution that respects both parties' needs.

The Role of Community and Social Connections In addition to individual relationships, community and social connections play a vital role in emotional well-being. Being part of a community provides a sense of belonging and support. Here's how to nurture social connections:

Join Groups and Activities: Participate in groups, clubs, or activities that align with your interests and values. Whether it's a sports team, book club, or volunteer organization, being involved in a community fosters social connections and provides opportunities for meaningful interactions.

Strengthen Family Bonds: Family relationships are often the foundation of social support. Make an effort to strengthen family bonds through regular communication, family gatherings, and shared activities. Show appreciation and support for your family members, and work together to overcome challenges.

Build a Support Network: Surround yourself with people who uplift and support you. A strong support network can provide emotional comfort, practical assistance, and valuable advice. Cultivate relationships with friends, mentors, colleagues, and other trusted individuals.

Balancing Relationships and Self-Care While nurturing positive relationships is important, it's also essential to balance them with self-care. Prioritize your own well-being and set boundaries to ensure that your relationships do not become overwhelming or draining. Here are some tips for balancing relationships and self-care:

Prioritize Self-Care: Make time for activities that recharge and rejuvenate you. Whether it's spending time alone, engaging in hobbies, or practicing mindfulness, prioritize self-care to maintain your emotional and mental well-being.

Communicate Your Needs: Openly communicate your needs and boundaries to others. Let them know when you need time for yourself or when you require support. Clear communication helps prevent misunderstandings and ensures that your needs are met.

Foster Independence: Encourage independence within your relationships. While support and connection are important, it's also essential to maintain a sense of autonomy and self-reliance. Foster a balance between togetherness and independence.

In conclusion, nurturing positive relationships is essential for emotional well-being and overall quality of life. By building trust, respect, and effective communication, and by practicing active listening, empathy, and conflict resolution, you can cultivate healthy and meaningful connections. Embrace the role of community and social connections, and balance relationships with self-care to enhance your emotional health. Prioritize positive relationships as a key aspect of your wellness journey and enjoy the benefits of a supportive and fulfilling life.

Does this cover it well? Ready to move on to the next chapter, or is there anything you'd like to adjust or discuss further?

Chapter 10: Integrative and Alternative Therapies

Understanding Integrative and Alternative Therapies

Summary: Define what integrative and alternative therapies are and how they differ from conventional medicine. Discuss the growing popularity and acceptance of these therapies in modern healthcare. Highlight the importance of evidence-based practices and the role of holistic approaches in promoting overall well-being.

Common Integrative Therapies

Summary: Explore common integrative therapies, such as acupuncture, chiropractic care, and massage therapy. Describe the principles behind each therapy, their benefits, and the conditions they are commonly used to treat. Provide examples of how these therapies can be integrated with conventional treatments to enhance patient outcomes.

Alternative Medicine Practices

Summary: Discuss alternative medicine practices, such as herbal medicine, homeopathy, and naturopathy. Explain the foundational concepts of these practices and their historical and cultural significance. Highlight the potential benefits and risks, and emphasize the importance of consulting with qualified practitioners.

Mind-Body Therapies

Summary: Examine mind-body therapies, such as meditation, yoga, and Tai Chi. Discuss how these practices promote mental, emotional, and physical health. Provide evidence of their effectiveness in managing stress, anxiety, and chronic pain. Highlight the importance of incorporating mind-body practices into daily routines for holistic wellness.

Integrating Therapies into Conventional Healthcare

Summary: Discuss the integration of integrative and alternative therapies into conventional healthcare settings. Highlight the role of healthcare providers in guiding patients through the use of these therapies. Provide examples of successful integrative healthcare programs and their impact on patient outcomes. Emphasize the importance of open communication and collaboration between patients and healthcare providers.

This outline covers the key aspects of integrative and alternative therapies, emphasizing their principles, benefits, and integration with conventional healthcare. Ready to dive into writing any of these points, or something else on your mind?

Integrative and alternative therapies have gained significant popularity in recent years as more individuals seek holistic approaches to health and well-being. These therapies offer complementary options to conventional medicine, focusing on the whole person—mind, body, and spirit. Understanding the principles and benefits of integrative and alternative therapies is essential for making informed decisions about incorporating them into your healthcare regimen.

Defining Integrative and Alternative Therapies Integrative therapies, also known as complementary therapies, are practices that are used in conjunction with conventional medical treatments to enhance overall health and well-being. These therapies aim to address not only the physical aspects of health but also the emotional, mental, and spiritual dimensions. Integrative medicine emphasizes a patient-centered approach, where the individual's unique needs and preferences are considered in the development of a comprehensive treatment plan.

Alternative therapies, on the other hand, are practices that are used in place of conventional medical treatments. These therapies often have roots in traditional healing practices and are based on holistic principles. While some alternative therapies lack extensive scientific validation, others have been studied and shown to provide benefits for certain conditions.

The Growing Popularity and Acceptance The growing popularity of integrative and alternative therapies can be attributed to several factors, including increased awareness of holistic health, dissatisfaction with conventional treatments, and a desire for more personalized healthcare options. Many individuals are seeking ways to take a proactive role in their health, and integrative therapies offer additional tools to support their wellness journey.

Healthcare institutions and practitioners are increasingly recognizing the value of integrative and alternative therapies. Many hospitals and clinics now offer integrative medicine programs that combine conventional treatments with complementary therapies such as acupuncture, massage, and meditation. This approach aims to provide comprehensive care that addresses the physical, emotional, and spiritual aspects of health.

Evidence-Based Practices While the popularity of integrative and alternative therapies continues to grow, it's essential to emphasize the importance of evidence-based practices. Evidence-based medicine involves using the best available research evidence to make informed decisions about patient care. For integrative and alternative therapies, this means evaluating the safety, efficacy, and potential benefits of these practices through rigorous scientific studies.

Not all integrative and alternative therapies have the same level of scientific validation. Some, such as acupuncture and mindfulness meditation, have been extensively studied and shown to provide benefits for specific conditions. Others may have limited research support, and their effectiveness may vary based on individual factors. It's important to approach these therapies with an open mind while also being critical and discerning about the available evidence.

Holistic Approaches to Health One of the key principles of integrative and alternative therapies is the focus on holistic health. Holistic health considers the whole person, recognizing that physical health is interconnected with emotional, mental, and spiritual well-being. This approach aims to promote balance and harmony within the individual, addressing the root causes of health issues rather than just treating symptoms.

Holistic health practices often emphasize prevention and self-care, encouraging individuals to take an active role in maintaining their well-being. This can include lifestyle modifications such as nutrition, exercise, stress management, and mindfulness practices. By addressing all aspects of health, holistic approaches aim to support long-term wellness and vitality.

The Role of Healthcare Providers Healthcare providers play a crucial role in guiding patients through the use of integrative and alternative therapies. Open communication between patients and providers is essential for developing a comprehensive treatment plan that incorporates both conventional and complementary approaches. Providers can help patients understand the potential benefits and risks of various therapies, ensuring that they make informed decisions about their health.

It's also important for healthcare providers to stay informed about the latest research and developments in integrative and alternative medicine. This knowledge allows them to offer evidence-based recommendations and support their patients in exploring holistic health options. Collaboration between conventional and integrative practitioners can lead to more effective and patient-centered care.

In conclusion, understanding integrative and alternative therapies involves recognizing their principles, benefits, and role in holistic health. These therapies offer valuable options for individuals seeking comprehensive and personalized approaches to well-being. By emphasizing evidence-based practices and fostering open communication with healthcare providers, individuals can make informed decisions about incorporating integrative and alternative therapies into their healthcare regimen. Embrace the potential of these therapies to enhance your overall health and wellness journey.

Common Integrative Therapies

Integrative therapies, also known as complementary therapies, are practices that work alongside conventional medical treatments to enhance overall health and well-being. These therapies focus on treating the whole person—mind, body, and spirit—by addressing various aspects of health. Here, we explore some of the most common integrative therapies, their principles, benefits, and the conditions they are commonly used to treat.

Acupuncture: Acupuncture is a key component of Traditional Chinese Medicine (TCM) that has been practiced for thousands of years. It involves the insertion of thin needles into specific points on the body, known as acupoints, to stimulate energy flow (Qi) and restore balance. According to TCM, Qi flows through pathways called meridians, and disruptions in this flow can lead to health issues. Acupuncture aims to correct these disruptions and promote the body's natural healing processes.

Benefits: Acupuncture is known for its effectiveness in managing pain, including chronic pain conditions such as arthritis, back pain, and migraines. It is also used to treat conditions such as anxiety, depression, digestive disorders, and menstrual irregularities. Acupuncture has been shown to improve overall well-being by reducing stress, enhancing relaxation, and boosting immune function.

Integration with Conventional Treatments: Acupuncture can be integrated with conventional treatments to enhance their effectiveness and reduce side effects. For example, cancer patients undergoing chemotherapy may use acupuncture to alleviate nausea, fatigue, and pain. It is essential to work with a qualified acupuncturist and communicate with your healthcare provider to ensure safe and effective integration.

Chiropractic Care Chiropractic care is a hands-on therapy that focuses on diagnosing and treating musculoskeletal disorders, particularly those related to the spine. Chiropractors use manual adjustments and manipulations to realign the spine and improve nervous system function. The underlying principle is that proper alignment of the musculoskeletal structure, particularly the spine, enables the body to heal itself without surgery or medication.

Benefits: Chiropractic care is widely used to treat back pain, neck pain, headaches, and joint issues. It can also improve posture, enhance mobility, and reduce the risk of future injuries. Chiropractic adjustments may provide relief for conditions such as sciatica, herniated discs, and sports injuries.

Integration with Conventional Treatments: Chiropractic care can complement conventional treatments by providing non-invasive pain relief and supporting overall musculoskeletal health. It is often used alongside physical therapy, pain management, and rehabilitation programs. Collaborating with both a chiropractor and a primary healthcare provider ensures comprehensive care and optimal outcomes.

Massage Therapy Massage therapy involves the manipulation of soft tissues, such as muscles, tendons, and ligaments, to promote relaxation, relieve pain, and enhance overall well-being. There are various types of massage, including Swedish massage, deep tissue massage, and sports massage, each with specific techniques and benefits.

Benefits: Massage therapy is known for its ability to reduce stress, anxiety, and muscle tension. It can alleviate pain from conditions such as fibromyalgia, chronic back pain, and sports injuries. Massage therapy also improves circulation, enhances lymphatic drainage, and supports the body's natural detoxification processes.

Integration with Conventional Treatments: Massage therapy can be used in conjunction with conventional treatments to enhance recovery and improve quality of life. For example, patients recovering from surgery or injury may benefit from massage therapy to reduce pain, improve mobility, and accelerate healing. It is important to communicate with your healthcare provider and massage therapist to ensure safe and effective integration.

Benefits of Integrative Therapies Integrative therapies offer several benefits, including:

Holistic Approach: Integrative therapies address the whole person, considering physical, emotional, mental, and spiritual aspects of health. This holistic approach promotes overall well-being and balance.

Complementary to Conventional Treatments: Integrative therapies can enhance the effectiveness of conventional treatments, reduce side effects, and improve patient outcomes. They provide additional tools for managing health conditions and supporting recovery.

Stress Reduction and Relaxation: Many integrative therapies, such as acupuncture and massage, promote relaxation and reduce stress. Stress reduction is essential for maintaining overall health and preventing chronic conditions.

Individualized Care: Integrative therapies often focus on personalized care, tailoring treatments to the individual's unique needs and preferences. This patient-centered approach fosters a sense of empowerment and active participation in one's health journey.

In conclusion, common integrative therapies such as acupuncture, chiropractic care, and massage therapy offer valuable benefits for enhancing overall health and well-being. These therapies can be integrated with conventional treatments to provide comprehensive care that addresses the whole person. By exploring and incorporating integrative therapies into your healthcare regimen, you can take a proactive approach to your wellness journey and enjoy the benefits of holistic health.

Alternative Medicine Practices

Alternative medicine practices encompass a wide range of therapies that are used in place of conventional medical treatments. These practices often have roots in traditional healing systems and are based on holistic principles that consider the whole person—mind, body, and spirit. Here, we explore some common alternative medicine practices, their foundational concepts, and their potential benefits and risks.

Herbal Medicine Herbal medicine, also known as botanical medicine or phytotherapy, involves using plant-based substances for therapeutic purposes. It is one of the oldest forms of medicine and has been used by various cultures worldwide. Herbal medicine relies on the medicinal properties of plants to prevent and treat diseases.

Foundational Concepts: Herbal medicine is based on the belief that plants contain natural compounds that can support the body's healing processes. Each plant has specific properties that can address different health issues. Herbalists use various parts of plants, such as leaves, flowers, roots, and bark, to create remedies in the form of teas, tinctures, capsules, and ointments.

Benefits: Herbal medicine is commonly used to support overall wellness and treat conditions such as digestive disorders, respiratory issues, skin problems, and stress. For example, peppermint is known for its digestive benefits, chamomile for its calming effects, and echinacea for its immune-boosting properties. Many people turn to herbal medicine for its natural approach and potential to reduce reliance on synthetic drugs.

Risks: While herbal medicine can offer benefits, it also carries risks, especially if used improperly. Some herbs can interact with medications or cause side effects. It is essential to consult with a qualified herbalist or healthcare provider before using herbal remedies, especially if you have underlying health conditions or are taking other medications.

Homeopathy: Homeopathy is a system of alternative medicine founded in the late 18th century by German physician Samuel Hahnemann. It is based on the principle of "like cures like," which suggests that substances that cause symptoms in healthy individuals can be used in diluted forms to treat similar symptoms in sick individuals.

Foundational Concepts: Homeopathy uses highly diluted substances prepared through a process called potentization. These remedies are believed to stimulate the body's vital force or healing energy. Homeopathic practitioners consider the individual's physical, emotional, and mental symptoms to select the appropriate remedy.

Benefits: Homeopathy is used to treat a wide range of conditions, including allergies, respiratory infections, digestive issues, and chronic pain. Some people turn to homeopathy for its gentle and non-invasive approach, as well as its focus on individualized treatment.

Risks: The efficacy of homeopathy is a subject of debate within the medical community. Critics argue that the extreme dilutions used in homeopathic remedies may render them ineffective, and scientific evidence supporting their efficacy is limited. It is important to approach homeopathy with an open mind while considering the available evidence and consulting with a qualified practitioner.

Naturopathy: Naturopathy, also known as naturopathic medicine, is a holistic approach to healthcare that emphasizes natural therapies and the body's inherent ability to heal itself. Naturopathy combines traditional healing practices with modern scientific knowledge.

Foundational Concepts: Naturopathy is based on principles such as the healing power of nature, identifying and treating the root cause of illness, and promoting preventive care. Naturopathic doctors (NDs) use a variety of therapies, including nutrition, herbal medicine, acupuncture, hydrotherapy, and lifestyle counseling.

Benefits: Naturopathy is used to address a wide range of health concerns, including chronic conditions, hormonal imbalances, digestive disorders, and mental health issues. Naturopathic doctors take a patient-centered approach, focusing on personalized care and addressing the underlying causes of illness.

Risks: While naturopathy offers a holistic approach to healthcare, it is important to ensure that treatments are evidence-based and provided by qualified practitioners. Some naturopathic therapies may lack rigorous scientific validation, and it is essential to communicate with both conventional and naturopathic healthcare providers to ensure safe and coordinated care.

Historical and Cultural Significance Many alternative medicine practices have deep historical and cultural roots. Traditional Chinese Medicine (TCM), Ayurveda, and Indigenous healing practices are examples of systems that have been used for centuries to promote health and well-being. These traditional practices are based on holistic principles and a deep understanding of the interconnectedness of mind, body, and spirit.

Consulting with Qualified Practitioners When exploring alternative medicine practices, it is crucial to consult with qualified practitioners who have the appropriate training and credentials. This ensures that treatments are safe, effective, and tailored to your individual needs. Qualified practitioners can provide guidance on the appropriate use of alternative therapies and help you make informed decisions about your health.

In conclusion, alternative medicine practices such as herbal medicine, homeopathy, and naturopathy offer holistic approaches to health and well-being. While these practices can provide benefits, it is important to consider their potential risks and consult with qualified practitioners. By exploring alternative medicine with an open mind and a critical eye, you can make informed decisions about incorporating these therapies into your healthcare regimen. Embrace the holistic principles of alternative medicine to support your overall health and wellness journey.

Mind-Body Therapies

Mind-body therapies are practices that focus on the connection between the mind and the body to promote holistic health and well-being. These therapies aim to improve mental, emotional, and physical health by using techniques that foster relaxation, mindfulness, and self-awareness. Here, we explore some common mind-body therapies, their benefits, and their effectiveness in managing stress, anxiety, and chronic pain.

Meditation: Meditation is a practice that involves focusing the mind and eliminating distractions to achieve a state of mental clarity and relaxation. There are various forms of meditation, including mindfulness meditation, loving-kindness meditation, and transcendental meditation, each with its unique techniques and benefits.

Benefits: Meditation is known for its ability to reduce stress and anxiety by calming the mind and promoting a sense of inner peace. Regular meditation practice can enhance emotional regulation, improve concentration, and boost overall mental well-being. It is also effective in reducing symptoms of depression and chronic pain.

Effectiveness: Numerous studies have shown that meditation can positively impact mental and physical health. Research indicates that mindfulness meditation can reduce the symptoms of anxiety disorders, improve sleep quality, and lower blood pressure. Brain imaging studies have also shown that meditation can increase gray matter density in areas associated with emotional regulation and self-awareness.

Incorporation into Daily Routine: To incorporate meditation into your daily routine, start with just a few minutes each day and gradually increase the duration. Find a quiet space, sit comfortably, and focus on your breath or a specific mantra. Consistency is key to reaping the benefits of meditation.

Yoga: Yoga is a mind-body practice that combines physical postures, breathing exercises, and meditation. Originating in ancient India, yoga aims to harmonize the mind, body, and spirit through various poses (asanas) and techniques.

Benefits: Yoga offers a wide range of benefits, including improved flexibility, strength, and balance. It also promotes relaxation, reduces stress, and enhances mental clarity. Yoga is effective in managing chronic pain conditions, such as lower back pain, and can improve overall physical health.

Effectiveness: Research has shown that yoga can reduce stress and anxiety, improve cardiovascular health, and enhance overall quality of life. Studies have found that regular yoga practice can lower cortisol levels, the body's primary stress hormone, and increase the production of endorphins, which promote feelings of well-being.

Incorporation into Daily Routine: To incorporate yoga into your daily routine, start with a few basic poses and gradually explore more advanced practices. Many online resources and classes are available to guide you. Dedicate a specific time each day for your practice to establish consistency.

Tai Chi Tai Chi, also known as Tai Chi Chuan, is a traditional Chinese martial art that involves slow, flowing movements and deep breathing. It is often described as "meditation in motion" due to its emphasis on mindfulness and relaxation.

Benefits: Tai Chi is known for its ability to improve balance, flexibility, and strength. It promotes relaxation, reduces stress, and enhances mental clarity. Tai Chi is also effective in managing chronic pain conditions, such as arthritis, and improving overall physical health.

Effectiveness: Research indicates that Tai Chi can improve balance and reduce the risk of falls in older adults. It also has positive effects on cardiovascular health, mental well-being, and immune function. Studies have shown that Tai Chi can reduce symptoms of anxiety and depression and improve overall quality of life.

Incorporation into Daily Routine: To incorporate Tai Chi into your daily routine, start with a few basic movements and gradually explore more complex forms. Many online resources and classes are available to guide you. Dedicate a specific time each day for your practice to establish consistency.

Integration with Conventional Healthcare Mind-body therapies can be integrated with conventional healthcare to enhance overall well-being and improve patient outcomes. These therapies provide additional tools for managing stress, anxiety, and chronic pain, complementing conventional treatments. Healthcare providers can guide patients in incorporating mind-body practices into their daily routines and offer resources for learning and practicing these therapies.

Holistic Wellness Mind-body therapies emphasize the importance of holistic wellness, recognizing the interconnectedness of mental, emotional, and physical health. By incorporating practices such as meditation, yoga, and Tai Chi into your daily routine, you can promote overall well-being and achieve a balanced and fulfilling life.

In conclusion, mind-body therapies such as meditation, yoga, and Tai Chi offer valuable benefits for enhancing mental, emotional, and physical health. These practices promote relaxation, reduce stress and anxiety, and improve overall well-being. By incorporating mind-body therapies into your daily routine and integrating them with conventional healthcare, you can take a holistic approach to your wellness journey and enjoy the benefits of a balanced and fulfilling life.

Integrating Therapies into Conventional Healthcare

Integrating integrative and alternative therapies into conventional healthcare settings is becoming increasingly common as more individuals seek holistic approaches to health and well-being. This integration aims to provide comprehensive care that addresses the physical, emotional, and spiritual aspects of health. By combining the best of both worlds, healthcare providers can enhance patient outcomes and promote overall wellness. Here's how integrative and alternative therapies can be successfully incorporated into conventional healthcare.

The Role of Healthcare Providers Healthcare providers play a crucial role in guiding patients through the use of integrative and alternative therapies. Open communication between patients and providers is essential for developing a comprehensive treatment plan that incorporates both conventional and complementary approaches. Providers can help patients understand the potential benefits and risks of various therapies, ensuring that they make informed decisions about their health.

Assessment and Personalization The integration of integrative and alternative therapies begins with a thorough assessment of the patient's health, lifestyle, and preferences. Healthcare providers work closely with patients to identify their specific needs and goals. This patient-centered approach ensures that the treatment plan is personalized and aligned with the individual's unique circumstances.

For example, a patient with chronic pain might benefit from a combination of conventional pain management techniques, such as medications and physical therapy, along with complementary therapies like acupuncture and massage therapy. By tailoring the treatment plan to the patient's needs, healthcare providers can offer a more holistic and effective approach to care.

Evidence-Based Integration While integrative and alternative therapies offer valuable benefits, it's essential to emphasize evidence-based practices. Healthcare providers should rely on scientific research and clinical evidence to guide the integration of these therapies. This ensures that treatments are safe, effective, and supported by credible data.

For instance, acupuncture has been extensively studied and shown to provide relief for chronic pain, migraines, and nausea. Mindfulness meditation has demonstrated effectiveness in reducing stress, anxiety, and depression. By incorporating therapies with a strong evidence base, healthcare providers can enhance patient outcomes and build trust in the integrative approach.

Successful Integrative Healthcare Programs Numerous healthcare institutions have developed successful integrative healthcare programs that combine conventional and complementary therapies. These programs offer valuable insights into the benefits of a holistic approach to care. Here are a few examples:

Integrative Oncology: Many cancer treatment centers have adopted integrative oncology programs that combine conventional treatments, such as chemotherapy and radiation, with complementary therapies like acupuncture, yoga, and nutritional counseling. These programs aim to reduce treatment-related side effects, improve quality of life, and support overall well-being for cancer patients.

Integrative Pain Management: Chronic pain management programs often incorporate integrative therapies to provide comprehensive care. These programs may include physical therapy, medications, acupuncture, massage therapy, and mindfulness practices. By addressing the physical and emotional aspects of pain, these programs help patients achieve better pain control and enhanced functioning.

Integrative Cardiology: Some cardiology centers offer integrative programs that combine conventional cardiac care with complementary therapies. These programs may include dietary counseling, stress management techniques, yoga, and acupuncture to support heart health and prevent cardiovascular disease. Integrative cardiology programs emphasize lifestyle modifications and holistic approaches to enhance cardiovascular wellness.

Collaborative Care Effective integration of integrative and alternative therapies requires collaboration and teamwork among healthcare providers. This collaborative care model involves various practitioners working together to provide comprehensive and coordinated care. For example, a patient's treatment team might include a primary care physician, a physical therapist, an acupuncturist, and a nutritionist. By sharing information and expertise, the team can develop a cohesive treatment plan that addresses all aspects of the patient's health.

Patient Education and Empowerment Educating patients about integrative and alternative therapies is essential for successful integration. Healthcare providers should offer resources and information to help patients make informed decisions about their treatment options. This includes explaining the potential benefits, risks, and evidence supporting various therapies.

Empowering patients to take an active role in their health is a key component of integrative care. Providers should encourage patients to ask questions, share their preferences, and participate in decision-making. By fostering a collaborative and supportive relationship, healthcare providers can enhance patient engagement and adherence to the treatment plan.

The Importance of Open Communication Open communication between patients and healthcare providers is critical for the successful integration of integrative and alternative therapies. Patients should feel comfortable discussing their interest in complementary therapies and any treatments they are currently using. Healthcare providers should listen to their patients' concerns, provide balanced information, and address any potential interactions or contraindications.

In conclusion, integrating integrative and alternative therapies into conventional healthcare settings offers a comprehensive approach to care that addresses the physical, emotional, and spiritual aspects of health. Healthcare providers play a crucial role in guiding patients through this integration, emphasizing evidence-based practices and personalized care. By fostering collaborative care, patient education, and open communication, healthcare providers can enhance patient outcomes and promote overall wellness. Embrace the potential of integrative and alternative therapies to support your health journey and achieve holistic well-being.

Chapter 11: Community and Support Systems

The Role of Community in Health and Wellness

Summary: Discuss the impact of community on individual health and wellness. Highlight the importance of a sense of belonging and social connection. Explain how communities provide emotional support, resources, and opportunities for social engagement. Provide examples of different types of communities, such as neighborhood groups, cultural organizations, and online forums.

Building Strong Support Systems

Summary: Explore the components of a strong support system, including family, friends, and professional networks. Discuss the importance of having diverse sources of support and how each can contribute to overall well-being. Provide strategies for building and maintaining strong support systems, such as regular communication, mutual support, and active participation in community activities.

The Benefits of Social Engagement

Summary: Examine the mental and physical health benefits of social engagement. Discuss how being actively involved in community activities can reduce stress, enhance mood, and improve overall health. Provide examples of social engagement activities, such as volunteering, group sports, and attending community events. Highlight the importance of finding activities that align with personal interests and values.

Overcoming Social Isolation

Summary: Address the issue of social isolation and its impact on health. Discuss the causes of social isolation, such as life transitions, geographical relocation, and health issues. Provide strategies for overcoming social isolation, including joining social groups, seeking professional help, and using technology to connect with others. Emphasize the importance of reaching out and staying connected.

Creating Inclusive Communities

Summary: Explore the importance of creating inclusive communities that welcome and support diverse individuals. Discuss the benefits of diversity and inclusivity for community health and well-being. Provide strategies for fostering inclusivity, such as promoting open dialogue, celebrating differences, and ensuring equal access to community resources. Highlight the role of community leaders and organizations in driving inclusivity initiatives.

This outline covers the essential aspects of community and support systems, emphasizing their role in health and wellness, the benefits of social engagement, strategies for overcoming social isolation, and the importance of inclusivity. Ready to dive into writing any of these points, or something else in mind?

Community plays a fundamental role in shaping individual health and wellness, offering a sense of belonging, social connection, and emotional support. Being part of a community provides individuals with resources, opportunities for social engagement, and a network of support that can positively impact their overall well-being. Understanding the importance of community in health and wellness helps highlight the need to foster and maintain strong social ties.

Sense of Belonging A sense of belonging is a vital aspect of emotional well-being. Being part of a community allows individuals to feel connected to others who share similar interests, values, or experiences. This connection fosters a sense of identity and purpose, reducing feelings of loneliness and isolation. Belonging to a community provides emotional security and a supportive environment where individuals can express themselves and feel understood.

Communities can take many forms, from neighborhood groups and cultural organizations to online forums and social clubs. Each type of community offers unique opportunities for connection and support. For example, neighborhood groups provide a local network of individuals who can offer assistance and companionship. Cultural organizations celebrate shared heritage and traditions, fostering a sense of pride and continuity. Online forums connect individuals with specific interests or challenges, providing a platform for shared experiences and advice.

Emotional Support Emotional support from a community is crucial for navigating life's challenges and maintaining mental health. Communities offer a safe space for individuals to share their feelings, seek advice, and receive encouragement. Whether it's through face-to-face interactions or virtual connections, the support of a community can help individuals manage stress, cope with difficulties, and build resilience.

For example, support groups for individuals dealing with specific health conditions, such as cancer or chronic pain, provide a network of people who understand their experiences and can offer empathy and practical advice. These groups create a sense of solidarity and reduce feelings of isolation, empowering individuals to face their challenges with greater strength and confidence.

Resources and Opportunities Communities often provide valuable resources and opportunities that contribute to individual health and wellness. These resources can include educational programs, recreational activities, healthcare services, and social events. Access to such resources enhances the quality of life and promotes a holistic approach to well-being.

Educational programs within communities offer information on various health topics, such as nutrition, exercise, mental health, and disease prevention. These programs empower individuals with knowledge and skills to make informed decisions about their health. Recreational activities, such as group fitness classes, sports leagues, and hobby clubs, encourage physical activity and social interaction, supporting both physical and mental health.

Healthcare services, such as community clinics, health screenings, and wellness workshops, provide accessible and affordable care for community members. Social events, such as festivals, gatherings, and celebrations, foster a sense of unity and joy, strengthening social bonds and enhancing emotional well-being.

Social Engagement Active participation in community activities promotes social engagement, which has numerous benefits for mental and physical health. Social engagement reduces stress, enhances mood, and improves cognitive function. Being involved in community activities provides a sense of purpose and fulfillment, encouraging individuals to stay active and engaged.

Examples of social engagement activities include volunteering, participating in group sports, attending community events, and joining clubs or organizations. Volunteering offers the opportunity to give back to the community, make a positive impact, and build meaningful connections. Group sports promote physical fitness, teamwork, and camaraderie. Community events, such as fairs, markets, and cultural celebrations, provide opportunities for socializing and enjoying shared experiences. Clubs and organizations, whether focused on hobbies, advocacy, or professional development, offer a platform for learning, collaboration, and friendship.

Types of Communities: Communities come in various forms, each offering distinct benefits and opportunities for connection:

Neighborhood Groups: Local communities where residents come together to address common concerns, support each other, and build a sense of belonging.

Cultural Organizations: Groups that celebrate shared heritage, traditions, and values, fostering cultural pride and continuity.

Online Forums: Virtual communities that connect individuals with specific interests, challenges, or goals, providing a platform for shared experiences and advice.

Social Clubs: Groups that bring people together based on common interests, hobbies, or activities, promoting social interaction and engagement.

Support Groups: Networks of individuals facing similar health conditions or life challenges, offering empathy, advice, and encouragement.

In conclusion, the role of community in health and wellness is multifaceted and essential for overall well-being. Communities provide a sense of belonging, emotional support, resources, and opportunities for social engagement. By fostering and maintaining strong social ties, individuals can enhance their quality of life and navigate life's challenges with greater resilience. Embrace the power of community and actively participate in the communities that resonate with you to support your health and wellness journey.

Building Strong Support Systems

A robust support system is a vital component of health and wellness, providing individuals with the emotional, social, and practical support needed to navigate life's challenges. A strong support system includes diverse sources of support, such as family, friends, and professional networks, each contributing to overall well-being in unique ways. Building and maintaining strong support systems requires intentional effort and active participation. Here's how to cultivate and sustain a network of support that enhances your quality of life.

Family Support Family is often the first and most enduring source of support. Family members provide emotional comfort, practical assistance, and a sense of belonging. They are typically the ones who know you best and can offer personalized support during difficult times. Here's how to strengthen family support:

Regular Communication: Maintain open and regular communication with family members. Share your thoughts, feelings, and experiences, and listen to theirs. Regular check-ins, whether through phone calls, video chats, or in-person visits, help maintain strong connections.

Mutual Support: Offer support to family members as well. Building a reciprocal relationship where both parties give and receive support fosters a sense of partnership and strengthens family bonds.

Shared Activities: Engage in activities that you enjoy together, such as family dinners, game nights, or outings. Shared experiences create lasting memories and reinforce family ties.

Friendship Networks Friends provide a different but equally important source of support. They offer companionship, empathy, and a sense of community. Friendships enrich our lives and contribute to emotional well-being. Here's how to cultivate and maintain strong friendships:

Invest in Relationships: Building strong friendships requires time and effort. Make an effort to reach out, plan activities, and stay connected with friends. Show genuine interest in their lives and be there for them in times of need.

Quality over Quantity: Focus on building deep and meaningful friendships rather than a large number of superficial connections. A few close friends who truly understand and support you are more valuable than numerous acquaintances.

Be Authentic: Authenticity is key to building trust and deepening friendships. Be yourself, share your true thoughts and feelings, and encourage your friends to do the same. Authenticity fosters genuine connections and mutual understanding.

Professional Networks Professional networks provide support in various aspects of life, including career development, education, and personal growth. These networks can include colleagues, mentors, coaches, and industry peers. Here's how to build and leverage professional support:

Networking: Actively participate in networking opportunities, such as conferences, workshops, and professional organizations. Building connections within your industry can open doors to new opportunities and provide valuable insights and advice.

Mentorship: Seek out mentors who can offer guidance, support, and feedback on your career and personal development. A mentor's experience and wisdom can help you navigate challenges and achieve your goals.

Collaboration: Foster collaborative relationships with colleagues and peers. Working together on projects, sharing knowledge, and supporting each other's growth can enhance your professional network and create a sense of community.

Diverse Sources of Support Having diverse sources of support is essential for overall well-being. Each type of support—family, friends, and professional networks—offers unique benefits and perspectives. A diverse support system ensures that you have access to a wide range of resources and people to turn to in different situations.

Strategies for Building and Maintaining Support Systems Building and maintaining strong support systems requires intentional effort and active participation. Here are some strategies to help you cultivate a robust network of support:

Be Present: Make an effort to be present and engaged in your relationships. Show genuine interest and attention to the people in your support system. Being present fosters deeper connections and mutual trust.

Offer Support: Support is a two-way street. Be willing to offer help, encouragement, and understanding to others. Building reciprocal relationships where support is given and received strengthens bonds and fosters a sense of partnership.

Stay Connected: Regular communication is key to maintaining strong support systems. Stay in touch through regular check-ins, messages, and social media. Make an effort to reach out, especially during significant life events or challenging times.

Participate in Community Activities: Engage in community activities, such as volunteering, attending events, and joining clubs or organizations. Active participation in community activities helps you meet new people, build connections, and expand your support network.

Seek Professional Help: Don't hesitate to seek professional help when needed. Therapists, counselors, and coaches can provide valuable support, guidance, and tools for personal growth and well-being.

The Impact of Strong Support Systems Strong support systems have a profound impact on health and wellness. They provide emotional comfort, practical assistance, and a sense of belonging. Having a robust network of support enhances resilience, reduces stress, and improves overall quality of life. Whether it's through family, friends, or professional networks, building and maintaining strong support systems is essential for navigating life's challenges and achieving well-being.

In conclusion, building strong support systems involves cultivating relationships with family, friends, and professional networks. Each source of support contributes to overall well-being in unique ways. By investing in relationships, offering mutual support, and actively participating in community activities, you can create a diverse and robust network of support that enhances your quality of life. Embrace the power of strong support systems and prioritize building and maintaining these connections as a key aspect of your health and wellness journey.

The Benefits of Social Engagement

Social engagement is a critical component of health and wellness, providing mental, emotional, and physical benefits. Being actively involved in community activities and maintaining strong social connections can enhance mood, reduce stress, and improve overall quality of life. Here's how social engagement contributes to well-being and ways to incorporate it into your daily routine.

Mental Health Benefits Active social engagement positively impacts mental health by reducing feelings of loneliness and isolation. When individuals participate in community activities and build social connections, they experience a sense of belonging and support. This social connectedness is essential for maintaining emotional stability and resilience.

Participating in social activities provides opportunities for positive interactions, which can uplift mood and enhance emotional well-being. Engaging in meaningful conversations, sharing experiences, and receiving empathy and understanding from others can alleviate symptoms of anxiety and depression. Social engagement also provides a distraction from negative thoughts and stressors, promoting a more balanced and positive outlook.

Physical Health Benefits Social engagement is linked to improved physical health outcomes. Individuals who are socially active tend to have lower levels of stress hormones, reduced inflammation, and stronger immune systems. Social interactions can buffer the effects of stress by providing emotional support and reducing the physiological impact of stressors.

Engaging in community activities often involves physical movement, such as walking, playing sports, or participating in group fitness classes. These activities promote physical fitness, increase energy levels, and support cardiovascular health. Social engagement encourages individuals to stay active and maintain a healthy lifestyle, reducing the risk of chronic conditions such as heart disease, obesity, and diabetes.

Cognitive Benefits Social engagement contributes to cognitive health by stimulating the mind and promoting mental agility. Participating in group activities, discussions, and cultural events challenges the brain and fosters cognitive functioning. Social interactions require communication, problem-solving, and memory recall, which help keep the mind sharp and engaged.

Research indicates that socially active individuals have a lower risk of cognitive decline and dementia. Engaging in intellectually stimulating activities, such as book clubs, educational workshops, and puzzles, supports brain health and enhances cognitive reserve. Social engagement provides a platform for lifelong learning and intellectual growth.

Examples of Social Engagement Activities There are numerous ways to incorporate social engagement into your daily routine. Here are some examples of activities that promote social connections and well-being:

Volunteering: Volunteering offers a sense of purpose and fulfillment while providing opportunities to connect with others. Whether it's helping at a local shelter, participating in environmental initiatives, or supporting community events, volunteering fosters social bonds and positive interactions.

Group Sports: Joining a sports team or participating in group fitness classes combines physical activity with social engagement. Team sports, such as soccer, basketball, or tennis, promote teamwork, camaraderie, and physical fitness. Group fitness classes, such as yoga, Pilates, or dance, provide a supportive environment for staying active and connected.

Community Events: Attending community events, such as festivals, fairs, and cultural celebrations, offers opportunities for socializing and enjoying shared experiences. These events provide a platform for meeting new people, exploring diverse cultures, and strengthening community ties.

Clubs and Organizations: Joining clubs or organizations that align with your interests and values fosters social connections and personal growth. Whether it's a book club, gardening group, or professional association, these clubs offer a sense of belonging and opportunities for collaboration and learning.

Support Groups: Participating in support groups for specific health conditions, life challenges, or personal interests provides a network of individuals who understand and empathize with your experiences. Support groups offer emotional comfort, practical advice, and a sense of solidarity.

Finding Activities that Align with Personal Interests To maximize the benefits of social engagement, it's important to find activities that align with your personal interests and values. Reflect on what brings you joy and fulfillment, and seek out opportunities that resonate with you. Here are some tips for finding the right activities:

Explore Your Interests: Identify hobbies, passions, and areas of curiosity. Whether it's art, sports, music, or community service, explore activities that align with your interests and bring you joy.

Try New Things: Be open to trying new activities and stepping out of your comfort zone. Experimenting with different social engagement opportunities can help you discover new passions and connections.

Seek Recommendations: Ask friends, family, or colleagues for recommendations on activities and events. They may have insights and suggestions that align with your interests and provide valuable social connections.

Use Technology: Utilize online platforms and social media to discover community activities, events, and groups. Many organizations and clubs have an online presence that makes it easy to find and join activities that interest you.

The Importance of Consistent Engagement Consistency in social engagement is key to reaping its benefits. Regular participation in community activities and maintaining social connections fosters a sense of routine and stability. Make social engagement a priority in your schedule and commit to staying actively involved.

In conclusion, social engagement offers numerous mental, emotional, and physical health benefits. Being actively involved in community activities and maintaining strong social connections enhances mood, reduces stress, and improves overall well-being. By finding activities that align with your interests, participating consistently, and seeking meaningful social interactions, you can enjoy the positive impact of social engagement on your health and quality of life. Embrace the opportunities for connection and fulfillment that social engagement provides and make it a central part of your wellness journey.

Overcoming Social Isolation

Social isolation is a growing concern with significant implications for health and well-being. It occurs when individuals have limited social interactions and feel disconnected from their community. Social isolation can lead to loneliness, mental health issues, and physical health problems. Understanding the causes of social isolation and implementing strategies to overcome it is essential for maintaining overall well-being.

Causes of Social Isolation Several factors can contribute to social isolation, including life transitions, geographical relocation, health issues, and societal changes. Here's a closer look at some common causes:

Life Transitions: Major life changes, such as retirement, the loss of a loved one, or becoming a caregiver, can lead to social isolation. These transitions often disrupt existing social networks and routines, making it challenging to maintain connections.

Geographical Relocation: Moving to a new city or country can be isolating, especially if individuals leave behind their established social networks. Building new connections in an unfamiliar environment can be daunting and take time.

Health Issues: Physical or mental health conditions can limit an individual's ability to engage in social activities. Chronic illness, mobility limitations, and mental health disorders such as anxiety and depression can contribute to feelings of isolation.

Societal Changes: Changes in societal norms and technology can impact social interactions. For example, the rise of remote work and online communication has altered traditional ways of socializing, sometimes leading to reduced face-to-face interactions.

Impact of Social Isolation on Health Social isolation can have severe consequences for both mental and physical health. Loneliness and social isolation are associated with increased risks of depression, anxiety, and cognitive decline. Physically, isolated individuals may experience higher levels of stress, inflammation, and a weakened immune system. Social isolation has been linked to an increased risk of chronic diseases such as heart disease, hypertension, and diabetes. Addressing social isolation is crucial for maintaining overall health and well-being.

Strategies for Overcoming Social Isolation Overcoming social isolation requires proactive efforts to build and maintain social connections. Here are some strategies to help individuals stay connected and engaged:

Join Social Groups: Participate in social groups, clubs, or organizations that align with your interests and values. Whether it's a book club, gardening group, or fitness class, joining social groups provides opportunities for meaningful interactions and friendships.

Volunteer: Volunteering offers a sense of purpose and fulfillment while providing opportunities to connect with others. Find volunteer opportunities in your community that resonate with your passions and skills. Volunteering can help you meet new people, give back to the community, and reduce feelings of isolation.

Attend Community Events: Participate in community events, such as festivals, fairs, and cultural celebrations. These events provide a platform for socializing and enjoying shared experiences. Attending community events fosters a sense of belonging and strengthens community ties.

Seek Professional Help: If social isolation is impacting your mental health, consider seeking professional help from a therapist or counselor. Mental health professionals can provide support, guidance, and strategies to cope with loneliness and build social connections.

Use Technology to Connect: Leverage technology to stay connected with friends and family, especially if geographical distance is a barrier. Video calls, social media, and online forums offer valuable platforms for maintaining relationships and engaging in social interactions. While online connections can't replace face-to-face interactions, they provide an essential means of staying connected.

Pursue Hobbies and Interests: Engage in activities and hobbies that bring you joy and fulfillment. Pursuing your passions can lead to new social connections with like-minded individuals. Whether it's painting, hiking, or playing music, participating in hobbies provides opportunities for social engagement and personal growth.

Reach Out: Don't hesitate to reach out to others and initiate social interactions. Sometimes, taking the first step to connect with someone can lead to meaningful relationships. Whether it's inviting a neighbor for coffee, joining a local group, or reconnecting with an old friend, reaching out fosters social connections.

Creating an Inclusive Environment Creating an inclusive environment that welcomes and supports diverse individuals is essential for addressing social isolation. Inclusive communities celebrate differences, promote open dialogue, and ensure equal access to resources and opportunities. Here are some strategies for fostering inclusivity:

Promote Open Dialogue: Encourage open and respectful conversations about diversity and inclusion. Creating a safe space for individuals to share their experiences and perspectives fosters understanding and empathy.

Celebrate Differences: Embrace and celebrate the unique qualities and contributions of individuals from diverse backgrounds. Recognizing and valuing diversity strengthens community bonds and promotes a sense of belonging.

Ensure Equal Access: Ensure that community resources, activities, and events are accessible to all individuals, regardless of their background, abilities, or socioeconomic status. Providing inclusive opportunities for participation helps reduce barriers to social engagement.

The Role of Community Leaders and Organizations Community leaders and organizations play a vital role in addressing social isolation and promoting inclusivity. They can implement initiatives that encourage social engagement, provide support, and create welcoming environments. Here are some examples of initiatives:

Social Programs: Develop and promote social programs that encourage community participation, such as social clubs, support groups, and recreational activities. These programs provide platforms for social interaction and support.

Outreach Initiatives: Implement outreach initiatives to connect with isolated individuals and offer resources and support. Outreach efforts can include home visits, phone check-ins, and providing information on available community services.

Inclusive Policies: Establish policies and practices that promote inclusivity and equal access. Ensure that community events, facilities, and services are designed to accommodate individuals with diverse needs and backgrounds.

In conclusion, overcoming social isolation is essential for maintaining overall health and well-being. By understanding the causes of social isolation and implementing strategies to build social connections, individuals can reduce loneliness and enhance their quality of life. Creating inclusive communities that celebrate diversity and promote open dialogue fosters a sense of belonging and support. Embrace the importance of social engagement and take proactive steps to stay connected and engaged in your community.

Creating Inclusive Communities

Creating inclusive communities is essential for promoting health and well-being. Inclusive communities welcome and support diverse individuals, ensuring everyone has equal access to resources, opportunities, and a sense of belonging. Embracing diversity and fostering inclusivity enhances community health, encourages social cohesion, and enriches the overall quality of life. Here's how to build inclusive communities and the benefits they bring.

The Importance of Inclusivity: Inclusivity is about creating an environment where all individuals, regardless of their background, abilities, or identities, feel valued, respected, and supported. Inclusive communities recognize and celebrate differences, fostering a culture of acceptance and understanding. Inclusivity is essential for several reasons:

Promotes Health and Well-being: Inclusive communities provide equitable access to healthcare, education, and social services, ensuring that everyone can achieve their full potential. Inclusivity reduces health disparities and improves overall community health.

Encourages Social Cohesion: Inclusivity fosters social connections and solidarity among community members. It creates a sense of unity and purpose, reducing social tensions and promoting harmony.

Enhances Quality of Life: Diverse and inclusive communities offer a rich tapestry of experiences, perspectives, and cultures. This diversity enriches the community, providing opportunities for learning, growth, and mutual respect.

Strategies for Fostering Inclusivity Building inclusive communities requires intentional efforts and a commitment to equity and diversity. Here are some strategies to promote inclusivity:

Promote Open Dialogue: Encourage open and respectful conversations about diversity, inclusion, and equity. Create safe spaces for individuals to share their experiences, perspectives, and concerns. Open dialogue fosters understanding, empathy, and mutual respect.

Celebrate Differences: Embrace and celebrate the unique qualities and contributions of individuals from diverse backgrounds. Organize cultural events, festivals, and activities that highlight the rich diversity of the community. Celebrating differences strengthens community bonds and promotes a sense of belonging.

Provide Equal Access: Ensure that all community resources, activities, and events are accessible to everyone. This includes making physical spaces accessible to individuals with disabilities, offering translation services, and providing affordable and inclusive programs. Equal access reduces barriers and promotes participation from all community members.

Implement Inclusive Policies: Establish policies and practices that promote inclusivity and equity. This includes anti-discrimination policies, inclusive hiring practices, and equitable resource allocation. Inclusive policies create a supportive environment where everyone feels valued and respected.

Engage Community Leaders: Community leaders and organizations play a crucial role in driving inclusivity initiatives. Engage leaders from diverse backgrounds to represent and advocate for their communities. Collaborative leadership ensures that the voices and needs of all community members are heard and addressed.

The Role of Community Organizations Community organizations are essential in promoting inclusivity and supporting diverse individuals. These organizations offer programs and services that address the unique needs of different community groups. Here's how community organizations can foster inclusivity:

Cultural Organizations: Cultural organizations celebrate the heritage and traditions of specific cultural groups, providing a sense of identity and belonging. These organizations offer cultural education, language classes, and cultural events that promote cross-cultural understanding.

Social Service Organizations: Social service organizations provide support and resources to individuals facing various challenges, such as poverty, homelessness, and domestic violence. By offering inclusive services, these organizations ensure that everyone has access to the help they need.

Advocacy Groups: Advocacy groups work to protect the rights and interests of marginalized and underrepresented communities. They advocate for policy changes, raise awareness of social issues, and promote equity and justice.

Benefits of Inclusive Communities Inclusive communities offer numerous benefits for individual and collective well-being:

Enhanced Social Support: Inclusivity fosters strong social networks and support systems, providing individuals with emotional and practical assistance. Social support is essential for mental health and resilience.

Increased Community Engagement: Inclusive communities encourage active participation and civic engagement. When individuals feel valued and included, they are more likely to contribute to community initiatives and volunteer efforts.

Improved Mental Health: Feeling accepted and supported within a community reduces feelings of loneliness and isolation. Inclusive communities promote mental health by creating a sense of belonging and connection.

Economic Growth: Diverse and inclusive communities attract businesses, talent, and investment. Economic growth is stimulated by the diverse perspectives, skills, and experiences that contribute to innovation and development.

In conclusion, creating inclusive communities is essential for promoting health, well-being, and social cohesion. By embracing diversity, fostering open dialogue, providing equal access, and implementing inclusive policies, communities can ensure that all individuals feel valued and supported. Community organizations and leaders play a vital role in driving inclusivity initiatives and supporting diverse populations. Embrace the principles of inclusivity and work towards building a community where everyone can thrive and enjoy a sense of belonging.

Chapter 12: Tailoring Wellness to Different Life S

Childhood and Adolescence

Summary: Discuss the unique wellness needs of children and adolescents. Highlight the importance of nutrition, physical activity, and mental health during these formative years. Provide guidance on establishing healthy habits early on and the role of parents and caregivers in supporting children's well-being. Emphasize the significance of regular check-ups, vaccinations, and developmental screenings.

Young Adulthood

Summary: Explore the wellness challenges and opportunities during young adulthood. Address the importance of maintaining a balanced diet, regular exercise, and mental health support as individuals transition to greater independence. Discuss the impact of lifestyle choices, such as alcohol consumption, smoking, and sleep patterns, on long-term health. Provide tips for managing stress and building resilience.

Midlife

Summary: Examine the wellness needs of individuals in midlife, including maintaining physical fitness, managing stress, and preventing chronic diseases. Discuss the importance of regular health screenings, such as cholesterol tests, blood pressure monitoring, and cancer screenings. Highlight strategies for achieving work-life balance, nurturing relationships, and pursuing hobbies and interests.

Older Adulthood

Summary: Focus on the wellness needs of older adults, including maintaining mobility, cognitive health, and social connections. Discuss the importance of bone health, fall prevention, and managing chronic conditions. Provide guidance on staying active, engaged, and connected with the community. Emphasize the role of regular medical check-ups, medication management, and mental health support.

Tailoring Wellness to Individual Needs

Summary: Highlight the importance of personalized wellness plans that take into account individual differences, such as genetics, health conditions, and personal preferences. Discuss the role of healthcare providers in creating tailored wellness strategies. Provide examples of personalized wellness interventions, such as custom exercise programs, dietary plans, and mental health support. Emphasize the importance of ongoing self-assessment and adjustments to maintain optimal well-being.

This outline covers the essential aspects of tailoring wellness to different life stages, emphasizing the unique needs and strategies for each stage. Ready to dive into writing any of these points, or something else in mind?

The formative years of childhood and adolescence are crucial for establishing the foundation of lifelong health and well-being. During these stages, the body and mind undergo significant growth and development, making it essential to prioritize wellness in all its dimensions. Tailoring wellness strategies to the unique needs of children and adolescents involves focusing on nutrition, physical activity, mental health, and regular medical care.

Nutrition Proper nutrition is fundamental for the growth and development of children and adolescents. A balanced diet provides the essential nutrients needed for physical and cognitive development, energy, and overall health. Here are some key nutritional guidelines for these age groups:

Balanced Meals: Ensure that children and adolescents consume a variety of foods from all food groups, including fruits, vegetables, whole grains, lean proteins, and healthy fats. Balanced meals provide the vitamins, minerals, and macronutrients needed for growth and development.

Hydration: Encourage regular water intake to maintain hydration. Water is essential for bodily functions, including temperature regulation, digestion, and nutrient transport. Limit sugary drinks, such as sodas and fruit juices, which can contribute to weight gain and dental issues.

Healthy Snacks: Offer nutritious snacks, such as fresh fruits, vegetables, yogurt, and nuts, to keep energy levels stable and support overall health. Avoid processed snacks high in sugar, salt, and unhealthy fats.

Physical Activity Regular physical activity is vital for the physical and mental well-being of children and adolescents. It promotes healthy growth, strengthens muscles and bones, improves cardiovascular health, and enhances mood and cognitive function. Here are some recommendations for promoting physical activity:

Daily Exercise: Aim for at least 60 minutes of moderate to vigorous physical activity each day. Activities can include playing sports, riding a bike, dancing, swimming, or simply playing outdoors.

Active Play: Encourage active play and reduce sedentary behaviors, such as excessive screen time. Active play fosters creativity, social skills, and physical fitness.

Family Involvement: Engage in physical activities as a family to set a positive example and make exercise a fun and enjoyable part of daily life.

Mental Health Mental health is as important as physical health during childhood and adolescence. Supporting mental well-being involves fostering a positive self-image, building resilience, and addressing any emotional or behavioral concerns. Here's how to support mental health:

Open Communication: Create an environment where children and adolescents feel comfortable expressing their thoughts and emotions. Encourage open and honest communication and actively listen to their concerns.

Stress Management: Teach stress management techniques, such as deep breathing, mindfulness, and relaxation exercises. Help them develop healthy coping mechanisms to handle stress and challenges.

Support Systems: Ensure that children and adolescents have access to supportive relationships with family members, friends, teachers, and mentors. Positive social connections provide emotional support and a sense of belonging.

Regular Medical Care Regular medical check-ups and screenings are essential for monitoring the health and development of children and adolescents. Preventive care helps identify and address any health issues early on. Here are some key aspects of regular medical care:

Vaccinations: Follow the recommended vaccination schedule to protect against infectious diseases. Vaccinations are crucial for preventing illnesses such as measles, mumps, rubella, and whooping cough.

Developmental Screenings: Regular developmental screenings assess physical, cognitive, and emotional development. Early identification of developmental delays or concerns allows for timely interventions and support.

Dental Care: Encourage good oral hygiene practices, such as regular brushing and flossing, and schedule regular dental check-ups to prevent cavities and maintain oral health.

Role of Parents and Caregivers Parents and caregivers play a pivotal role in supporting the health and well-being of children and adolescents. Here are some ways they can contribute:

Healthy Role Models: Set a positive example by practicing healthy habits, such as eating nutritious foods, staying active, and managing stress. Children often emulate the behaviors of their caregivers.

Education and Guidance: Educate children about the importance of nutrition, physical activity, and mental health. Provide guidance and support in making healthy choices and developing lifelong wellness habits.

Safe and Nurturing Environment: Create a safe, nurturing, and supportive home environment that fosters physical, emotional, and mental well-being. Ensure that children have access to healthy foods, opportunities for physical activity, and a supportive network of family and friends.

In conclusion, childhood and adolescence are critical stages for establishing the foundation of lifelong health and well-being. By focusing on proper nutrition, regular physical activity, mental health support, and preventive medical care, we can support the healthy development of children and adolescents. Parents and caregivers play a vital role in guiding and nurturing their well-being, helping them build healthy habits that will benefit them throughout their lives. Embrace the opportunity to support the wellness of children and adolescents and empower them to thrive and reach their full potential.

Young Adulthood

Young adulthood is a transformative stage characterized by greater independence and new responsibilities. During this period, individuals establish patterns and habits that can influence their long-term health and well-being. Tailoring wellness strategies to the unique challenges and opportunities of young adulthood involves focusing on nutrition, physical activity, mental health, and lifestyle choices.

Nutrition Maintaining a balanced diet is crucial for supporting the energy levels and physical health of young adults. During this stage, individuals often face busy schedules, academic or work commitments, and social activities, which can impact their eating habits. Here are some key nutritional guidelines for young adults:

Balanced Diet: Aim to consume a variety of nutrient-dense foods from all food groups, including fruits, vegetables, whole grains, lean proteins, and healthy fats. Balanced meals provide essential vitamins, minerals, and macronutrients needed for overall health.

Hydration: Stay hydrated by drinking plenty of water throughout the day. Water is essential for maintaining bodily functions, including digestion, circulation, and temperature regulation. Limit the intake of sugary drinks and excessive caffeine.

Meal Planning: Plan and prepare meals in advance to avoid relying on fast food or processed snacks. Meal prepping can save time and ensure access to healthy, homemade meals even on busy days.

Physical Activity Regular physical activity is essential for maintaining physical fitness, reducing stress, and supporting mental well-being. Here are some recommendations for promoting physical activity during young adulthood:

Exercise Routine: Aim for at least 150 minutes of moderate-intensity aerobic exercise per week, such as brisk walking, running, cycling, or swimming. Include strength training exercises at least two days a week to build and maintain muscle mass.

Active Lifestyle: Incorporate physical activity into daily routines, such as walking or biking to work, taking the stairs instead of the elevator, and engaging in active hobbies like hiking or dancing.

Social Engagement: Participate in group sports or fitness classes to combine physical activity with social interaction. Exercising with friends or joining a sports team can make workouts more enjoyable and provide motivation and accountability.

Mental Health Mental health is a critical aspect of overall well-being during young adulthood. This period often involves significant life changes, such as transitioning to higher education, starting a career, and building relationships. Supporting mental health involves managing stress, building resilience, and seeking support when needed. Here are some strategies for maintaining mental health:

Stress Management: Develop healthy coping mechanisms for managing stress, such as mindfulness meditation, deep breathing exercises, and physical activity. Identify and address stressors early to prevent them from becoming overwhelming.

Resilience Building: Cultivate resilience by setting realistic goals, maintaining a positive mindset, and learning from setbacks. Building resilience helps individuals navigate challenges with greater ease and confidence.

Social Support: Maintain strong social connections with family, friends, and peers. Social support provides emotional comfort, reduces feelings of isolation, and enhances overall well-being. Don't hesitate to seek professional help from a therapist or counselor if needed.

Lifestyle Choices Lifestyle choices during young adulthood can have a significant impact on long-term health. Making informed decisions about alcohol consumption, smoking, sleep patterns, and other behaviors is essential for maintaining overall well-being. Here are some tips for making healthy lifestyle choices:

Alcohol Consumption: If you choose to drink alcohol, do so in moderation. The Centers for Disease Control and Prevention (CDC) defines moderate drinking as up to one drink per day for women and up to two drinks per day for men. Excessive alcohol consumption can lead to health issues such as liver disease, cardiovascular problems, and mental health disorders.

Smoking Cessation: If you smoke, quitting is one of the most important steps you can take to improve your health. Smoking is a leading cause of preventable diseases, including cancer, heart disease, and respiratory conditions. Seek support from healthcare providers, smoking cessation programs, and support groups to help you quit.

Sleep Patterns: Prioritize good sleep hygiene to ensure adequate rest and recovery. Aim for 7-9 hours of sleep per night. Establish a regular sleep schedule, create a relaxing bedtime routine, and minimize exposure to screens and stimulants before bedtime.

Managing Stress and Building Resilience Managing stress and building resilience are essential for navigating the challenges of young adulthood. Here are some additional strategies to support these efforts:

Time Management: Develop effective time management skills to balance academic, work, and social commitments. Create a schedule that allows for productive work, relaxation, and self-care. Prioritize tasks, set realistic goals, and avoid overcommitting.

Self-Care: Practice self-care by engaging in activities that bring you joy and relaxation. Self-care can include hobbies, spending time in nature, reading, or practicing mindfulness. Taking time for yourself helps recharge and maintain overall well-being.

Financial Wellness: Develop healthy financial habits, such as budgeting, saving, and managing debt. Financial stress can impact mental health, so learning to manage finances responsibly is crucial for long-term well-being.

The Role of Healthcare Providers Regular medical check-ups and preventive care are essential for maintaining health during young adulthood. Healthcare providers can offer valuable guidance on nutrition, exercise, mental health, and lifestyle choices. Here are some key aspects of regular medical care:

Health Screenings: Schedule regular health screenings, such as cholesterol tests, blood pressure monitoring, and sexually transmitted infection (STI) screenings. Early detection and intervention are crucial for preventing and managing health issues.

Vaccinations: Stay up-to-date with recommended vaccinations, including the HPV vaccine, flu vaccine, and any other vaccines recommended by your healthcare provider.

Mental Health Support: Don't hesitate to seek mental health support from a therapist or counselor if needed. Mental health professionals can provide valuable tools and strategies for managing stress, building resilience, and maintaining emotional well-being.

In conclusion, young adulthood is a transformative stage with unique wellness challenges and opportunities. By prioritizing nutrition, physical activity, mental health, and making informed lifestyle choices, young adults can establish healthy habits that support long-term well-being. Regular medical care and the guidance of healthcare providers are essential for navigating this stage with confidence and maintaining overall health. Embrace the journey of young adulthood and take proactive steps to build a balanced and fulfilling life.

Midlife

Midlife is a dynamic phase marked by a range of experiences, from career advancements and family responsibilities to personal growth and self-discovery. During this stage, individuals often juggle multiple roles, making it essential to prioritize wellness to maintain physical, emotional, and mental health. Tailoring wellness strategies to the unique needs of midlife involves focusing on physical fitness, stress management, preventive health care, and nurturing relationships.

Physical Fitness Maintaining physical fitness during midlife is crucial for overall health and well-being. As the body ages, metabolic rate slows down, muscle mass decreases, and the risk of chronic conditions increases. Here are some key strategies for promoting physical fitness during midlife:

Regular Exercise: Engage in at least 150 minutes of moderate-intensity aerobic exercise per week, such as brisk walking, jogging, swimming, or cycling. Include strength training exercises at least two days a week to build and maintain muscle mass, improve bone density, and boost metabolism.

Flexibility and Balance: Incorporate flexibility and balance exercises, such as yoga and Tai Chi, to enhance mobility, prevent falls, and reduce the risk of injuries. These practices also promote relaxation and mental clarity.

Active Lifestyle: Stay active throughout the day by incorporating physical activity into daily routines. Take the stairs instead of the elevator, walk or bike to work, and engage in active hobbies like gardening or dancing.

Stress Management Midlife often comes with increased responsibilities and stressors, such as managing a career, caring for family members, and planning for retirement. Effective stress management is essential for maintaining emotional and mental well-being. Here are some strategies for managing stress:

Mindfulness and Meditation: Practice mindfulness and meditation to reduce stress and enhance emotional resilience. Mindfulness involves paying attention to the present moment without judgment, while meditation promotes relaxation and mental clarity. Regular practice can help manage stress and improve overall well-being.

Time Management: Develop effective time management skills to balance work, family, and personal commitments. Create a schedule that allows for productive work, relaxation, and self-care. Prioritize tasks, set realistic goals, and avoid overcommitting.

Self-Care: Engage in activities that bring joy and relaxation, such as reading, spending time in nature, or pursuing hobbies. Self-care helps recharge and maintain overall well-being. Make time for yourself and prioritize self-care as an essential part of your routine.

Preventive Health Care Regular health screenings and preventive care are vital for detecting and addressing health issues early. Preventive care helps manage risk factors and prevent chronic diseases. Here are some key aspects of preventive health care during midlife:

Health Screenings: Schedule regular health screenings, such as cholesterol tests, blood pressure monitoring, diabetes screenings, and cancer screenings (e.g., mammograms, colonoscopies, and prostate exams). Early detection and intervention are crucial for preventing and managing health issues.

Vaccinations: Stay up-to-date with recommended vaccinations, including the flu vaccine, shingles vaccine, and any other vaccines recommended by your healthcare provider. Vaccinations help protect against infectious diseases and support overall health.

Bone Health: Pay attention to bone health by getting regular bone density screenings, especially for women at risk of osteoporosis. Include calcium-rich foods and vitamin D in your diet to support bone health. Weight-bearing exercises, such as walking and resistance training, also help strengthen bones.

Nurturing Relationships Strong social connections and supportive relationships play a significant role in overall well-being during midlife. Building and maintaining healthy relationships with family, friends, and colleagues enhance emotional and mental health. Here are some ways to nurture relationships:

Quality Time: Spend quality time with loved ones and engage in meaningful activities together. Whether it's family dinners, weekend outings, or shared hobbies, quality time strengthens bonds and fosters a sense of belonging.

Effective Communication: Maintain open and honest communication with family, friends, and colleagues. Active listening, expressing thoughts and feelings, and showing empathy and understanding are key components of effective communication.

Mutual Support: Offer and seek support within your relationships. Building reciprocal relationships where both parties give and receive support fosters a sense of partnership and strengthens connections.

Pursuing Hobbies and Interests Midlife is an excellent time to explore new hobbies and interests or rekindle old ones. Pursuing activities that bring joy and fulfillment enhances overall well-being and provides a sense of purpose. Here are some tips for pursuing hobbies and interests:

Explore New Activities: Be open to trying new activities and stepping out of your comfort zone. Whether it's painting, learning a musical instrument, or taking up a new sport, exploring new interests can bring excitement and growth.

Join Clubs and Groups: Participate in clubs, organizations, or groups that align with your interests and values. Joining social groups provides opportunities for connection, learning, and collaboration.

Set Personal Goals: Set personal goals related to your hobbies and interests. Having goals provides a sense of direction and motivation, helping you stay engaged and committed to your activities.

Work-Life Balance Achieving a healthy work-life balance is essential for maintaining overall well-being during midlife. Balancing career responsibilities with personal and family life requires intentional effort and effective time management. Here are some strategies for achieving work-life balance:

Set Boundaries: Establish clear boundaries between work and personal life. Define specific work hours and avoid bringing work-related tasks into personal time. Setting boundaries helps prevent burnout and allows for quality time with loved ones.

Delegate Responsibilities: Don't hesitate to delegate responsibilities at work and home. Sharing tasks with colleagues, family members, and friends lightens the load and fosters a sense of teamwork and collaboration.

Take Breaks: Schedule regular breaks throughout the day to rest and recharge. Taking short breaks can enhance productivity and reduce stress. Plan vacations or time off to unwind and relax.

In conclusion, midlife is a dynamic phase with unique wellness needs and opportunities for personal growth. By prioritizing physical fitness, managing stress, engaging in preventive health care, nurturing relationships, and pursuing hobbies and interests, individuals can maintain overall well-being during this stage. Achieving work-life balance and practicing self-care are essential for navigating the challenges and opportunities of midlife with confidence and fulfillment. Embrace the journey of midlife and take proactive steps to build a balanced and enriching life.

Older Adulthood

Older adulthood is a stage of life that brings unique wellness needs and opportunities for maintaining health, vitality, and independence. As individuals age, prioritizing wellness becomes increasingly important for preserving physical and cognitive health, managing chronic conditions, and staying socially connected. Tailoring wellness strategies to the needs of older adults involves focusing on mobility, cognitive health, social engagement, and preventive care.

Maintaining Mobility Maintaining mobility is crucial for independence and overall quality of life in older adulthood. Regular physical activity helps preserve muscle strength, flexibility, and balance, reducing the risk of falls and injuries. Here are some key strategies for promoting mobility:

Regular Exercise: Engage in regular physical activity, including aerobic exercises such as walking, swimming, and cycling, to support cardiovascular health and overall fitness. Aim for at least 150 minutes of moderate-intensity aerobic exercise per week.

Strength Training: Include strength training exercises at least two days a week to build and maintain muscle mass and bone density. Use resistance bands, free weights, or bodyweight exercises like squats and push-ups.

Flexibility and Balance: Practice flexibility and balance exercises, such as yoga, Tai Chi, or stretching routines, to enhance mobility and prevent falls. These practices also promote relaxation and mental clarity.

Cognitive Health Supporting cognitive health is essential for maintaining mental sharpness and quality of life in older adulthood. Cognitive decline is not inevitable, and there are strategies to keep the mind active and engaged. Here's how to support cognitive health:

Mental Stimulation: Engage in activities that challenge the brain, such as puzzles, reading, learning new skills, or playing musical instruments. Mental stimulation promotes cognitive function and neuroplasticity.

Social Engagement: Stay socially active by participating in community events, joining clubs, or engaging in group activities. Social interactions provide mental stimulation and emotional support, reducing the risk of cognitive decline.

Healthy Diet: Consume a balanced diet rich in nutrients that support brain health, such as omega-3 fatty acids, antioxidants, and vitamins. Include foods like fatty fish, berries, nuts, and leafy greens in your diet.

Adequate Sleep: Prioritize good sleep hygiene to ensure adequate rest and cognitive function. Aim for 7-9 hours of sleep per night and establish a regular sleep schedule.

Social Connections Maintaining social connections is vital for emotional well-being and overall health in older adulthood. Strong social ties provide emotional support, reduce feelings of loneliness, and enhance quality of life. Here are some ways to stay socially connected:

Community Involvement: Participate in community activities, such as volunteering, attending social events, or joining clubs and organizations. Community involvement fosters a sense of belonging and purpose.

Family and Friends: Maintain regular communication with family and friends through phone calls, video chats, or in-person visits.

Building and nurturing relationships provide emotional comfort and support.

Support Groups: Join support groups for specific health conditions, life challenges, or interests. Support groups offer a network of individuals who understand and empathize with your experiences, providing valuable advice and encouragement.

Preventive Care Regular medical check-ups and preventive care are essential for managing health and preventing chronic conditions in older adulthood. Preventive care helps detect and address health issues early, reducing the risk of complications. Here are some key aspects of preventive care:

Health Screenings: Schedule regular health screenings, such as blood pressure monitoring, cholesterol tests, diabetes screenings, and cancer screenings (e.g., mammograms, colonoscopies). Early detection and intervention are crucial for managing health conditions.

Vaccinations: Stay up-to-date with recommended vaccinations, including the flu vaccine, shingles vaccine, and pneumonia vaccine. Vaccinations help protect against infectious diseases and support overall health.

Bone Health: Pay attention to bone health by getting regular bone density screenings, especially for those at risk of osteoporosis. Include calcium-rich foods and vitamin D in your diet to support bone health. Weight-bearing exercises, such as walking and resistance training, also help strengthen bones.

Managing Chronic Conditions Many older adults live with chronic conditions that require ongoing management and care. Effective management of chronic conditions is essential for maintaining quality of life and preventing complications. Here's how to manage chronic conditions effectively:

Medication Management: Take medications as prescribed and keep an updated list of all medications. Communicate with healthcare providers about any side effects or concerns. Use tools such as pill organizers or medication reminders to ensure adherence.

Regular Monitoring: Monitor health metrics, such as blood pressure, blood sugar levels, and weight, regularly. Keep track of any changes and report them to healthcare providers. Regular monitoring helps manage conditions and detect any issues early.

Healthy Lifestyle: Adopt a healthy lifestyle that includes a balanced diet, regular physical activity, and stress management. Healthy habits support overall well-being and improve the management of chronic conditions.

Staying Active and Engaged Staying active and engaged in life is essential for emotional, mental, and physical well-being in older adulthood. Here are some ways to stay active and engaged:

Hobbies and Interests: Pursue hobbies and interests that bring joy and fulfillment. Whether it's gardening, painting, or playing music, engaging in activities that you love enhances quality of life.

Lifelong Learning: Continue learning and exploring new interests. Take classes, attend workshops, or participate in educational programs. Lifelong learning stimulates the mind and promotes cognitive health.

Travel and Exploration: If possible, travel and explore new places. Travel provides opportunities for adventure, learning, and social interactions. Whether it's a local day trip or an international vacation, exploring new environments enriches life experiences.

The Role of Healthcare Providers Healthcare providers play a crucial role in supporting the wellness of older adults. Regular medical care, personalized treatment plans, and ongoing support are essential for maintaining health and well-being. Here are some key aspects of the role of healthcare providers:

Comprehensive Care: Provide comprehensive care that addresses physical, emotional, and mental health. Develop personalized treatment plans that consider individual needs and preferences.

Patient Education: Educate patients about their health conditions, treatment options, and preventive care. Empower patients to take an active role in managing their health.

Support and Resources: Offer support and resources for managing chronic conditions, maintaining mobility, and staying socially connected. Connect patients with community services, support groups, and educational programs.

In conclusion, older adulthood is a stage with unique wellness needs and opportunities for maintaining health, vitality, and independence. By focusing on maintaining mobility, supporting cognitive health, staying socially connected, and engaging in preventive care, older adults can enhance their quality of life. Effective management of chronic conditions, staying active, and seeking regular medical care are essential for navigating this stage with confidence and fulfillment. Embrace the journey of older adulthood and take proactive steps to build a balanced and enriching life.

Tailoring Wellness to Individual Needs

Everyone's wellness journey is unique, influenced by factors such as genetics, health conditions, personal preferences, and lifestyle. Tailoring wellness strategies to individual needs is essential for achieving optimal health and well-being. Personalized wellness plans take into account these differences and provide customized interventions that align with each person's goals and circumstances. Here's how to create and implement personalized wellness plans and the importance of ongoing self-assessment.

Personalized Wellness Plans Personalized wellness plans are designed to address the specific needs and goals of an individual. These plans consider various factors, including medical history, current health status, genetic predispositions, lifestyle, and personal preferences. Here's how to create a personalized wellness plan:

Comprehensive Assessment: Start with a comprehensive assessment of the individual's health, including medical history, current health conditions, dietary habits, physical activity levels, and mental health. Assessing these factors provides a baseline for developing a personalized plan.

Set Specific Goals: Identify specific, measurable, achievable, relevant, and time-bound (SMART) goals that align with the individual's health and wellness objectives. Goals may include weight management, improving fitness, managing stress, or enhancing overall well-being.

Customized Interventions: Develop customized interventions that address the individual's unique needs. These interventions may include dietary plans, exercise programs, stress management techniques, and mental health support. Tailor each intervention to fit the person's lifestyle and preferences.

Role of Healthcare Providers Healthcare providers play a crucial role in creating and implementing personalized wellness plans. They offer expert guidance, support, and resources to help individuals achieve their health goals. Here's how healthcare providers contribute to personalized wellness:

Medical Expertise: Healthcare providers use their medical expertise to assess health risks, diagnose conditions, and recommend appropriate interventions. They consider the individual's medical history, current health status, and genetic predispositions when developing a wellness plan.

Collaborative Approach: Providers work collaboratively with individuals to set realistic goals and create a personalized plan. They take into account the person's preferences, lifestyle, and values, ensuring that the plan is practical and achievable.

Ongoing Support: Healthcare providers offer ongoing support and monitoring to track progress, adjust interventions, and address any challenges. Regular check-ins and follow-up appointments ensure that the wellness plan remains effective and aligned with the individual's goals.

Examples of Personalized Wellness Interventions Personalized wellness interventions can vary widely based on individual needs and goals. Here are some examples of customized interventions:

Custom Exercise Programs: Develop an exercise program tailored to the individual's fitness level, preferences, and goals. For example, a person with joint issues may benefit from low-impact exercises like swimming or yoga, while someone aiming to build muscle may focus on strength training.

Dietary Plans: Create a dietary plan that aligns with the individual's nutritional needs, health conditions, and preferences. For example, a person with high cholesterol may follow a heart-healthy diet rich in fiber, omega-3 fatty acids, and lean proteins. A person with food allergies may need a specialized plan that avoids specific allergens.

Mental Health Support: Provide personalized mental health support based on the individual's needs. This may include therapy, counseling, mindfulness practices, or stress management techniques. Tailor the support to address specific mental health concerns, such as anxiety, depression, or stress.

Chronic Condition Management: Develop a personalized plan for managing chronic conditions, such as diabetes, hypertension, or arthritis. This may include medication management, lifestyle modifications, regular monitoring, and support from healthcare providers.

Importance of Ongoing Self-Assessment Ongoing self-assessment is essential for maintaining and adjusting personalized wellness plans. Regular self-assessment helps individuals track their progress, identify areas for improvement, and make necessary adjustments to stay on track. Here's how to conduct ongoing self-assessment:

Monitor Progress: Keep track of progress towards wellness goals by recording health metrics, such as weight, blood pressure, fitness levels, and mental health. Use journals, apps, or tracking tools to document progress and identify patterns.

Reflect on Experiences: Reflect on your experiences and how the wellness plan is working for you. Consider what is going well, what challenges you are facing, and what changes may be needed to improve the plan's effectiveness.

Adjust Goals: Be flexible and open to adjusting goals as needed. As you make progress, you may set new goals or modify existing ones to reflect your evolving needs and priorities.

Seek Feedback: Seek feedback from healthcare providers, fitness trainers, nutritionists, or mental health professionals. Their insights and expertise can help you make informed decisions about adjusting your wellness plan.

Adapting to Life Changes Life is dynamic, and wellness plans should be adaptable to changing circumstances. Personal and environmental factors, such as job changes, family responsibilities, health conditions, or aging, can impact your wellness journey. Here's how to adapt your wellness plan to life changes:

Stay Flexible: Be open to modifying your wellness plan as needed to accommodate new challenges and opportunities. Flexibility ensures that your plan remains relevant and effective.

Prioritize Self-Care: During times of change, prioritize self-care to maintain your well-being. Self-care helps you manage stress, stay resilient, and navigate transitions with greater ease.

Reassess and Realign: Periodically reassess your wellness goals and strategies to ensure they align with your current situation and priorities. Realigning your plan keeps you focused and motivated.

In conclusion, tailoring wellness to individual needs involves creating personalized plans that address unique health conditions, preferences, and goals. Healthcare providers play a crucial role in developing and supporting personalized wellness strategies. Ongoing self-assessment and adaptability are essential for maintaining and adjusting wellness plans to achieve optimal health and well-being. Embrace the principles of personalized wellness and take proactive steps to create a plan that supports your unique journey towards a balanced and fulfilling life.

www.ingramcontent.com/pod-product-compliance
Lightning Source LLC
Chambersburg PA
CBHW020334160726
47992CB00004B/1844